Nutrition from Earth and Cosmos

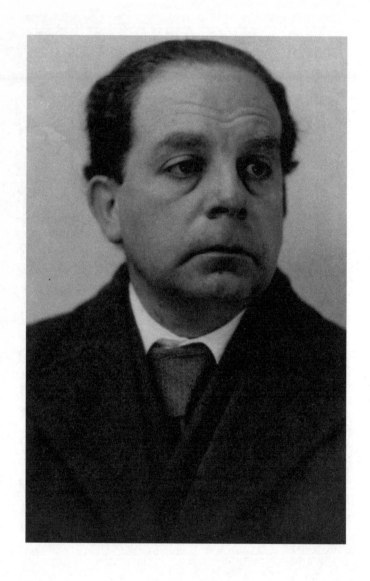

Nutrition from Earth and Cosmos

Karl König

Floris Books

Karl König Archive Publication, Vol. 15
Subject: Agriculture, science
Series editor: Richard Steel

Karl König's collected works are issued by
the Karl König Archive, Aberdeen
in co-operation with the Ita Wegman Institute
for Basic Research into Anthroposophy, Arlesheim

Edited and translated by Carlotta and James Dyson

First published in this form in German as *Irdische und kosmische Ernährung*
by Verlag Freies Geistesleben in 2011
First published in English by Floris Books in 2015

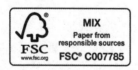

MIX
Paper from
responsible sources
FSC
www.fsc.org
FSC® C007785

British Library CIP Data available
ISBN 978-178250-163-3

Printed in Great Britain
by Bell & Bain, Glasgow

Contents

The Meteorological Organs

Lectures for farmers at Botton Hall, Yorkshire, 1958

Two Essays

A Note About this Volume

Richard Steel

The current volume is designed to provide some insight into Karl König's concerted endeavours over many decades to achieve a deeper understanding of the question of nutrition, both with regard to the qualitative significance of foodstuffs, and to the process of nutrition itself. Of course we hear the voice of the physician, as well as the therapeutic educator and the founder of communities. Yet König's elaborations are integral to a holistic healing impulse: he is concerned not only with the way our food is grown but with the very healing of the earth itself; this is for him a social task and one that needs to be connected with a renewed Christian impulse; the task constitutes no less than a modern Christianisation of the earth itself. This concern was directly linked to the work he had already begun in Silesia in the 1930s, when a new school for a comprehensive approach to social work was founded with the cooperation of priests of the Christian Community.[1]

This gave rise to the first challenge in connection with the publication of these texts, as König's most penetrating courses on these questions had been for farmers, on whom he had placed high expectations and great demands regarding content. This relationship with the farmers was of such importance to König that he always expected his medical colleagues to attend the agricultural conferences. In the invitation to the 1943

7

conference we detect a certain 'exclusivity', which the organisers (the Biodynamic Agricultural Association in Clent, UK) had particularly welcomed (see facsimile on pp. 12–13). In addition to Karl König, contributors included Walter Johannes Stein, Ernst Lehrs, Dr Alfred Heidenreich (one of the founders of the Christian Community and senior priest in Britain) while Emil Roth, father of Camphill co-founders Alix and Peter, introduced discussions around practical questions.

Three of the lecture cycles included in this volume were given at agricultural conferences: The Cultural Impulse of Agriculture in 1943, The Streams of Cosmic and Earthly Nutrition in 1953 and The Meteorological Organs of the Earth and of the Human Being in 1958. For Karl König these two topics – nutrition and agriculture – were so closely connected that this forms a companion volume to Social Farming. However, as the boundaries between the two are not easily delineated, this volume contains much that should be of interest to farmers; the 1943 course was known among the farmers of the old Camphill School as the 'Milk Course'. It follows from this that considerable background knowledge was assumed, including a certain amount of specialist medical knowledge and independent work with anthroposophy. Would-be participants in the conference of 1958 were actually expected to have studied Rudolf Steiner's lectures on Introducing Anthroposophical Medicine.

Generally speaking, König expected quite a lot of his audience, as the aim of the lectures was not the transmission of detailed expert knowledge, but the development of an imaginative overview of the scientific facts, guiding the listener to a new level of understanding and individual research transcending professional expertise. He wanted to build interdisciplinary bridges, capable of stimulating new directions in individual study and research that would at the same time engender new dimensions in community building.

From 1959 onwards, particularly through the collaboration with Lieven Blockhuys, the work with farmers took a different direction, as engagement with the social question and the healing of the earth came more to the fore. Lectures focussing more closely on these aspects have therefore been included in the volume *Social Farming*.

Apart from the short working text from 1964 and his essay on grace before meals, König was not able to edit the texts in this volume himself. However, we know that he was very thorough in preparing any of his own lectures or writings for publication – the few lectures of his that he did manage to revise bear witness to this. Apart from the lectures in Prague, which were held in German, in his British sojourn he was obliged to use a language that he never completely mastered. Although he was lecturing in English as early as 1929 and his listeners were able to follow him with interest and enthusiasm, there are reports from the 1960s, referring to 'quite a peculiar English'. This fact presented challenges for the note-takers at the time, as it does for present-day editors. Fortunately the Archive contains his preparatory notes for most conferences and individual lectures, which König usually wrote in German. Unfortunately we also have to contend with illegible passages and damaged manuscripts. This applies to the Prague manuscripts, which miraculously survived König's various journeys fleeing the Nazi regime.

Carlotta and James Dyson have not only translated the German texts (including the introductory essays) but have significantly contributed to the editing process. Thanks are also due to Professor Reinhold Fäth, who has reconstructed most of the drawings, and to those who have helped to prepare these texts with their professional expertise. Collecting and preparing this volume with these colleagues has been a very lively and exciting process. This is surely the way König would have wished his work to be dealt with – to be regarded not as results but rather as a catalyst for ever new research, for ever renewed enthusiasm for the mysteries of existence and for ever more fruitful collaboration among human beings. I hope that this book can make further contributions in this spirit.

About the English Edition
James and Carlotta Dyson

Everything that Richard Steel has written applies comprehensively to this new and revised English publication, which has been based on the texts of the 2011 German edition. However, those texts that are transcripts of lectures originally given in English have been thoroughly re-edited from the English original (the 1953 and 1958 lectures were previously published as *Earth and Man*), with a view to rendering them in as acceptable and contemporary an English style and idiom as is compatible with their informal style of delivery. We have not simply translated König's lecture transcripts, but have checked them for factual accuracy on the basis of other archive material as well as current scientific and medical knowledge. No attempt has been made to sanitise their content or expression for its own sake. As translators/editors of the English edition, and in the spirit of the original English editors of *Earth and Man* (Carlo Pietzner, Alix Roth and Peter Roth), we have exercised 'a certain responsibility in the development of [our own] judgment and care' in judiciously modifying the reports of statements made by Karl König, endeavouring to do this in a way he himself might have done if he had been faced with the task of preparing the texts for publication in the twenty-first century.

The sole aim has been to clarify as far as reasonably possible the considerable number of ambiguities that they contain, as well as to adjust the linguistic and stylistic irregularities that frequently obscured their meaning. This would particularly affect the reader unfamiliar either with Steiner's anthroposophy or with basic standard medical physiology.

Where there has been serious ambiguity or unclarity, we have attempted to revise the wording in a way as close to what we intuit Karl König was intending to convey, on the basis of our own interpretation. Occasionally we have inevitably had to bridge gaps and rely on our personal understanding and judgment, and obviously cannot guarantee that the results are always beyond question. Hopefully, however, our collaboration has gone a long way to combining the best of our individual abilities, namely those of basic medical knowledge, familiarity with general anthroposophy and with Steiner's medical lectures in particular, as well as linguistic skills both in English and German. (Carlotta's first language is German; James's is English.)

From

DERYCK J. DUFFY

Home Farm, Clent Grove

CLENT, STOURBRIDGE
WORCS.

Telephone .. .. Hagley 253

Station .. .. Hagley, G.W.R.

HEATHCOT HOUSE,

BLAIRS,

ABERDEEN.

8th Sept. 1943.

My dear Dr. Konig,

    I am sending you herewith a brief lay-out for the little conference on October 12th.

    I am arranging for people like Glentanar, Wilson, Ellis and others practising the methods to attend for "closed talks". I think this will give us an opportunity to speak without reserve on the use of artificials and sprays. I have made the headings for the actual lectures rather general in character, so you will be able to go for them without reserve and say whatever you wish without having regard to members of the public being present.

    Mrs. Mayo and my wife will bring the children over on Saturday afternoon at four o'clock as you have suggested.

        Kindest regards,

            Yours sincerely,

The invitation to the 'Closed Conference' at Heathcot House, Oct 12–18, 1943.

HEATHCOT HOUSE,
BLAIRS, ABERDEENSHIRE

ONE WEEK CONFERENCE: OCTOBER 12th - 18th, 1943.

ABOUT FIFTEEN PERSONS interested in the agricultural indications of Rudolf
Steiner, are invited to attend this meeting, which will be in the form of
a 'Closed Conference'. This will enable lecturers to discuss present day
problems from many angles, and pass on information obtained in private
talks with Rudolf Steiner. By limiting the number attending, ample
opportunity will occur for questions and discussions.
THE GENERAL THEME will be The Cultural Impulse behind Agriculture. General
lectures on this theme will he held in the mornings (10 a.m.) except Tuesdq
12th, to allow for the arrival of guests, when the first lecture will be
held at 4.30 p.m.; and evenings (7.15. p.m.) Afternoon sessions will be
arranged each day according to weather. Talks will be given by Mr. E.Roth
on farm buildings, and other practical issues will be discussed.

G E N E R A L   L E C T U R E S

OCT-OBER	MORNING	AFTERNOON	EVENING
12th	———	An historical survey of Agriculture, from Initiate Knowledge to Science, Dr.W.J.Stein.	Continuation - Dr. W.J.Stein.
13th	Continuation - Dr. W.J.Stein.	To be arranged	Natural Science and Spiritual Science - Dr. E. Lehrs.
14th	Continuation - Dr. E.Lehrs.	" "	Continuation - Dr. E .Lehrs.
15th	The food we produce and its effect on Man. Assimilation and digestion. Health and Disease. Dr. K.Konig	" "	Continuation - Dr. K. Konig.
16th	Continuation - Dr. K.Konig.	" "	A Summary: Dr.W.J.Stein, Dr. E.Lehrs, Dr. K.Konig.
17th	Christian Community Service in Aberdeen.	" "	The Mystery of Substance Dr. A. Heydenreich.
18th	General discussion of the practical issues involved.		

VISITORS may arrive on Monday 11th, or on the morning of Tuesday 12th.
Will they please bring emergency ration cards, including points.

Nutrition and Healing

Erdmut Schädel

Karl König had the gift of impressively penetrating subjects from virtually all walks of life and conveying this to others. He was able to address people of all kinds, whether professionals or laymen, provided they were open to a spiritual world view. His deepest concern was always to speak out of the spiritual conception of the human being as developed by Rudolf Steiner in his many writings and lectures. This also applies to the field of nutrition. Today, fifty to sixty years after König's lectures and seminars on this subject were given, this topic is being widely debated out of a growing recognition that human health depends on it. However, the perspective from which it is viewed is of critical importance.

If we regard foods merely as products of the different substances and elements, we will be led more and more into an analytic approach, which ultimately bears no relationship to the true source of nourishment. Ever more substances, trace elements, etc., are being discovered, and their harmful, pathogenic effects described. For almost every substance a pathogenic, carcinogenic effect can be identified as soon as it is removed from its natural context and is no longer an integral part of the whole. By themselves, processes in nature have a destructive effect on the human organism if they are introduced directly into the metabolism, without first being prepared in the right way.

15

The more precisely the metabolic processes controlled by enzymes are analysed, the more we lose sight of the whole. A clockwork mechanism that has been dismantled will never again produce a functioning clock unless the higher principle of its design has been understood. Similarly, in the modern science of nutrition the connection between nature and the cosmos, between microcosm and macrocosm, is more and more being lost.

This is precisely the interrelationship that König was addressing in his lectures and seminars on nutrition. He repeatedly stresses the fact that foods merely serve as media for quite other qualities that live in the food and are active in the human organism. These qualities cannot be quantified, cannot be measured, analysed or assessed according to calorific values or units of energy; they are of a much more subtle character, and their mode of action is still largely hidden from our outer senses. During the process of nutrition an actual process of metabolism (literally, a complete change or overthrow) takes place, during which the food is divested of its substance, which is essentially toxic to the human organism, leaving only the actual formative process that stands behind the substance.

It was thoughts such as these, derived from the spiritual research of Rudolf Steiner, that Karl König presented in a lively and down-to-earth manner to the most diverse groups of people such as physicians, therapeutic educators, nurses, farmers and mothers, giving practical indications right down to details of the choice of particular foods and food preparation.

At a time when food is judged according to the efficiency of the substances and to calorific balance, prepared in as short a time as possible (fast food), and also consumed hurriedly, it may be opportune and worthwhile to reconsider Karl König's thoughts and perspectives on this subject. The passage of time has not diminished their relevance; they point to an attitude that transcends the mere consumption of food. What comes to expression in these lectures is that we 'do not live by bread alone,' but that through the intake of food we are re-connected to forces which create a whole out of the parts. This process corresponds to a healing process, through which the human being is again connected to the whole of the cosmos.

Erdmut Schädel is a paediatrician at the Ita Wegman Clinic in Arlesheim, Switzerland. After attending the Waldorf School in Wuppertal, Germany, he trained in curative education at the Sonnenhof in Arlesheim, and then studied medicine and paediatrics in Germany. He has published books on child development.

131) The _Ahrimanic_ beings are of an etheric,
the _Luciferic_ ones of an astral nature.
Michael defeats the Ahrimanic powers.
Raphael heals the Luciferic forces.

132) _Kidney stones_ are essentially _lenses,_
being formed in the eye of the kidney.
The kidney is becoming too much of a sense organ,
thereby coming under the influence of the crystallising forces.
Gall stones are emergent otoliths [ear stones].
Here the same applies, on a different level.

133) More and more frequently I discover that women
suffering from _myomas_ [fibroids] or who have _breast cancer_
have in their life never given birth.
The forces of the embryonic period metamorphose
and become peculiarities that are only
able to receive growing life but not ensouled life.

134) In contemplating the difference between
a _foodstuff_ and a _medicine_
the following guidelines can be applied:
For foodstuffs it is important that they are demolished
and lose all their particular qualities, so that in their place
the cosmic nutrition stream can take effect.
In a medicine it is important that just their particular properties

131.) Die ahrimanischen Wesen sind ätherischer,
die luziferischen, astralischer Natur.
Michael besiegt die ahrimanischen Mächte.
Raphael heilt die luziferischen Kräfte.

‡

132.) Nierensteine sind nichts anderes, als
sich bildende Linsen im Nieren-Auge.
Die Niere wird zu stark Sinnesorgan & unter-
liegt dadurch den kristallisierenden Kräften.
Gallensteine sind sich bildende Otholiten.
Hier liegt das gleiche, auf anderer Stufe vor.

‡

133.) Immer öfter finde ich, dass Frauen, die
an Myomen leiden oder ein Mamma-Ca
haben in ihrem Leben niemals geboren
haben. Die Kräfte der Embryonalzeit verwandeln sich & werden zu Absonderlichkeiten
die nur wachsendes, aber nicht beseeltes
Leben erzeugen.

‡

134.) Beim Bedenken des Unterschiedes zwischen
einem Nahrungsmittel & einem Heilmittel
kommt folgende Übersicht: Beim Nahrungsmittel ist es notwendig, dass dieses zerschlagen
wird & alle Eigenkräfte verliert, damit an
seiner Stelle der kosmische Ernährungsstrom
wirksam werden kann.
Beim Heilmittel muss gerade die Eigen-

About foods and medicines. Notebook entry of 1932

19

*are preserved, thereby stimulating the awakening of
the human being's own soul forces.
Spices and fragrances form a kind of transition.
Remedies, however, have to be prepared in such a way that
their own essential properties can work within the organism.
Through them the world enters the human being. Therefore
it is only possible to heal outside of the middle region,
because breathing is inserted into the body as part of the
macrocosm (25920 [Platonic Year])!
Remedies enter the organism not in order to be
transformed, but in order to transform!
This means that nutritional power can be transformed into
healing power when something from the lower part of the
organism is lifted up into the higher organism.
The true image of this is the Last Supper,
from where the power of nutrition flows the healing of the
world.*

*Here a being takes the whole world into himself
as a pure mirror. The world becomes man,
man becomes world. This is the highest form of healing,
Only from there can <u>grace</u> then flow.*

wirksamkeit erhalten bleiben, damit die Eigen-seel-
ischen Kräfte des Menschen an ihm erwach.

Den Übergang bilden die Gewürze & Düfte.

Heilmittel müssen also so zubereitet werden, daß
ihre Eigenkräfte im Organismus wirken können. Die
Welt tritt mit ihnen in den Menschen ein. Deshalb
kann nur über das mittlere System hinweg geheilt
werden, weil die Atmung eingebaut ist in den
Leib als ein Teil des Makrokosmos (25 9 20)!

Heilmittel gehen in den Organismus, nicht um
verwandelt zu werden, sondern um zu verwandeln!

Deshalb kann Nahrungskraft in Heilkraft verwandelt
werden, wenn aus der unteren Organisation etwas
in die obere Organisation hinaufgehoben wird.

Das reale Bild dafür ist das heilige Abendmahl,
wo aus der Kraft der Nahrung, das Teil der Welt
erfließt.

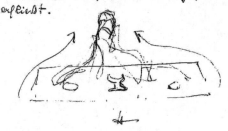

Hier nimmt ein Wesen die ganze Welt in sich
hinein als reiner Spiegel. Die Welt wird Mensch,
der Mensch wird Welt. Das ist die höchste Heilung.
Nur daraus kann dann _Gnade_ fließen.

About foods and medicines. Notebook entry of 1932

Anthroposophic Nutritional Research

Petra Kühne

Rudolf Steiner first started lecturing on nutrition well over one hundred years ago. Later on, particularly in the last years of his life, he would make reference to this theme, for example in his courses on education for special needs and on agriculture as well as in lecture cycles for physicians and teachers. As Steiner never gave a lecture cycle specifically devoted to nutrition, his indications are scattered across other cycles and courses, and have had to be carefully assembled and correlated. Steiner's approach to nutrition differed markedly from the one current at the time. For him the human being was a spiritual as well as a physical being, whose nutrition needed to take into account both these components. This runs counter to modern scientific nutritional science with its materialistic view of nutrients. In the 1920s Steiner increasingly developed his picture of 'nutrition through the senses' complementing the idea of nutrition as ordinarily understood. He described how foods were largely destroyed through digestion, only to be completely rebuilt within the human body. His statement that foods do not supply the human body with the substances necessary for its up-building, but that essentially they induce an inner activity within the body, constituted a big challenge at the time and to a large extent still does to this day.

Only much later in the twentieth century did biochemical discoveries relating to cellular and energy metabolism as well as
the sequence of processes in cellular respiration make Steiner's
statements more comprehensible.

From indications to a science of nutrition

In the eighty-five years since Steiner's death, how has the picture of nutrition that he presented been further researched? We
can look at this period from the point of view of thirty-three
year rhythms; three times thirty-three constitutes roughly
one hundred years. After one hundred years it becomes clear
whether an impulse such as this has been able to find a place
in culture and has become established. In the first phase the
idea is taken up and disseminated. With respect to Steiner's
indications on nutrition these first thirty-three years run from
1924 to 1957. This coincides essentially with the activity of
Karl König. His lectures published in this volume were all held
during this period. Karl König himself said in the first lecture
in Thornbury in 1953 (pp. 161f):

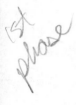

> To begin with ... until 1935, we were simply
> enthusiastic. We went out into the world proclaiming
> the threefold nature of man, the cosmic and earthly
> nutrition streams ... We were too confident ... We
> gradually discovered how in fact all that Rudolf Steiner
> said in the course of the years on one or another subject
> fits together bit by bit until a more or less complete
> picture has been developed; only this picture is so
> tremendous that one is hardly able to comprehend it all
> at once.

This phase entailed the gathering together of all Steiner's
nutritional indications as well as further work to develop a comprehensive and coherent picture of an anthroposophic concept
of nutrition. The publication of Steiner's lectures took place in

stages; the sifting of the material was in itself a research and study project, to which several people devoted their energies.

Ehrenfried Pfeiffer (1899–1961) collaborated with Rudolf Steiner as a young man; a chemist by training, he devoted the whole of his working life to researching the qualities of food, developing ways of picturing etheric (life) forces, and promoting an understanding of the principles of biodynamic agriculture. He emigrated to the United States in the 1930s where he lectured extensively on nutrition. Pfeiffer was in contact with König, as both were working in English-speaking countries. Pfeiffer was one of the frequent visitors to Pilgramshain where research into biodynamic methods was done, meeting König there between 1929 and 1933. There were other physicians besides König who concerned themselves with nutrition. Among them was *Eugen Kolisko* (1893–1939), who knew König from Vienna. He was the first school doctor at the Stuttgart Waldorf School, and, like König, had to emigrate to Britain. Kolisko arrived in England in 1935, but suffered an early death there in 1939. His wife *Lili Kolisko* (1889–1976) developed the copper chloride crystallisation research method. *Werner Christian Simonis* (1898–1984) was also a colleague of König's. He was the author of several books in German based on the anthroposophic conception of nutrition and designed to make anthroposophy intelligible for the layman and applicable to everyday living. The chemist *Rudolf Hauschka* (1891–1969), founder of the Wala pharmaceutical company, also occupied himself with questions of nutrition. He too was in contact with Karl König. His book *Nutrition,* as well as those by Simonis, were the first steps of research, collating the many indications on nutrition given by Rudolf Steiner.

In this way a concept of nutrition evolved, suitable for presentation to a wider public. Hauschka as well as König and Pfeiffer endeavoured to corroborate anthroposophic insight with the latest findings of scientific research. Hauschka, for example, incorporated vitamin research into his books and even developed a classification system of vitamins in relation to the four elements.

(The term vitamin was first coined in 1912 for Thiamin. Vitamin C was not isolated from lemon juice until 1931). König's work on nutrition has remained virtually unknown, though Hauschka, in *Nutrition,* provided a glimpse into his ideas, reprinting König's description of hormones and the processes by which substances are built up. Hauschka was aware of the fact that the hormones, which had only recently been investigated scientifically, played a key role in the realm of life processes, and that König had developed a classification system based on his own original ideas.

Nutrition research and nutrition courses

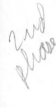

The second thirty-three-year period from 1957 to 1990 began with a group of younger physicians of the new generation, who felt the need to take hold of the original ideas in a different way. This second phase is devoted to implementation and experimentation. In 1955 the physician *Gerhard Schmidt* (1908–90) established a laboratory to research medical aspects of nutrition, using copper chloride crystallisation, at the Goetheanum in Dornach, Switzerland. In 1960 the House of Nutrition (now Crystallisation Laboratory) was built for this purpose. In 1963 he took on the leadership of the Agriculture Section, extending it into the Section for Agriculture and Nutrition. In collaboration with his colleague *Udo Renzenbrink* (1913–94), nutritional experiments were carried out, researching the different grains and their effect on the human being. This was rather novel; Karl König had not been concerned with different grains. Apart from the grains used in the making of bread, and locally, barley and oats, other kinds of grains were hardly given any consideration.

This was also the era of the first nutrition conferences and the publication of the magazine *Beiträge zu einer geisteswissenschaftlichen Ernährungshygiene.* This Section activity ceased in 1970. Udo Renzenbrink started a working group for nutritional research in Bad Liebenzell, Germany, in which he pursued his grain research, disseminating his results in numerous courses and seminars. It was in the course of this work that the seven

26

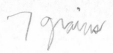

grains were seen to be linked to the seven planets and the seven days of the week. During this time the nutritional impulse was strengthened in many institutions. The utilisation of the different grains according to the seven days of the week – often erroneously attributed to Rudolf Steiner – became established in Waldorf kindergartens and schools. In 1980 an Association for the Promotion of Healthy Nutrition in Community Settings was founded in Germany with the aim of promoting anthroposophic nutrition and its principles more vigorously in the institutions.

In association with the ecological and whole food movement, there was a growing interest in nutrition from an anthroposophic perspective. During this time anthroposophic nutrition was viewed as one of the alternative schools of nutrition and there was even some scientific interest shown. During this time Gerhard Schmidt published his books and held regular lectures and seminars on nutrition. Further research topics included the importance of heat in nutrition, which arose in response to the spread of the raw food movement and the advocacy of uncooked grains in nutrition, as well as diets and nutritional therapy. 'Nutrition through the senses'– often also called 'cosmic nutrition' – was another topic, but this remained very much confined to Steiner's indication and as yet showed little reworking. The reason for this seems to lie in the sheer power of Steiner's images which to this day remain hard to understand. Here Karl König's contributions certainly have the potential to help move things forward.

Image-generating methods were increasingly employed in nutrition research. Elisabeth Hälsig (1924–90) investigated a large number of foodstuffs by means of capillary dynamolysis in order to capture and make visible the forces engendering growth and form in plants. A research group under the auspices of the Natural Science Section investigated the possibilities and limitations of this method.

At the end of the 1980s there was a change. Interest in cookery courses diminished. This not only affected anthroposophical circles but also the curricula of other educational establishments. A certain phase had run its course. A standard of wholefood nutrition had, however, been established and organic produce supplemented the foods on offer. Biodynamic agriculture was now a recognised part of the ecological movement. This standard became incorporated in legislation in the European Union in 1991.

Achieving cultural impact

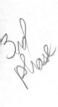

During this new phase, interest in nutrition shifted from consumers to experts. This third phase of the hundred year period will show whether the original ideas have achieved cultural impact, whether they have become integrated into the culture and have established connections with existing 'teachers' or ideas. In the 1990s a new generation brought with it new tasks. The 'wholegrain wave' receded, and the importance of vegetables for the supply of secondary plant substances was recognised. Yet the talk was still of vital *substances* rather than vital *forces;* that is, the search was for material substances having specific effects. More and more experts recognised the great influence of nutrition on health. Nutritional advice and therapy increasingly became available. Yet there was also a realisation that a nutritional approach offering only knowledge of nutrients did not produce the desired results because human nutritional behaviour is a lot more multidimensional. The inclusion of psychological methods came to be seen as important.

This also provided an entry point for anthroposophic nutrition, which consistently takes its starting point from an individual approach to nutrition, based on the anthroposophic conception of the human being. At the same time, Asian teachings such as Ayurvedic nutrition (from India) or traditional Chinese nutrition became increasingly important. Hildegard nutrition (after Hildegard von Bingen, 1098–1179) was rediscovered and spread. What these older forms of nutrition have in common with anthroposophic nutrition is the fact that they are based on different or more comprehensive principles than those of natural science: they include the concept of forces, and are based on a broader conception of the human being. Anthroposophic nutrition goes even further in that it takes account of the significance of substances and their spiritual origin. It was only due to natural science that the significance of the mere substances came into the foreground. Karl König addresses this topic in his lectures, particularly in those of 1953.

The nutritional studies of different foodstuffs, such as meat or grains, and their effect on human beings, which Gerhard Schmidt and Udo Renzenbrink had started, was extended by research in which the variable was merely the nutritional quality of the food. In a study of nutritional quality in 2005 a number of nuns in a convent were given food which for a certain period of time was of biodynamic quality and for a further period of time of conventional quality. This study was carried out by Karin Huber under the auspices of the Forschungsring für biologisch-dynamische Wirtschaftsweise (Research Group for Biodynamic Agriculture) under the leadership of Nikolai Fuchs.[1]

Since 1998 the Arbeitskreis für Ernährungsforschung (Research Group for Nutrition) has researched such topics as nutrition through the senses and developing the capacity for perception of the quality of foodstuffs. The centre also offers advanced training in anthroposophic nutrition.

Within the anthroposophic institutions the demands of communal catering led to questions of nutrition and food quality: Why Demeter and organic foods? What is the situation with regard to grain dishes? How do we evaluate modern catering systems? Processes have started that engage with contemporary issues in order to discover and establish an individual profile.

We are therefore seeing an interest in nutrition in society, and this in turn enables anthroposophic nutrition to contribute its own ideas. In this context it is important to emphasise that the aim is not to promote an alternative nutrition movement from the early twentieth century, whose relevance is confined to that period, but to demonstrate that these ideas are capable of contributing to the solution of nutritional problems of the present and the future. Viewed from this perspective, it would appear to be an opportune moment for Karl König's lectures on nutrition to be published, as a stimulus for renewing creative interest in this field.

Petra Kühne is leader of the Arbeitskreis für Ernährungsforschung (Research Group for Nutrition) in Bad Vilbel, Germany. She is a nutritionist with a PhD in agricultural science. She is editor of the journal Ernährungsrundbrief *and holds courses and lectures as well as contributing to publications on nutrition.*

Cosmic and Earthly Nutrition: a Topical Question

Anita Pedersen

This volume is a companion to *Social Farming,* the volume on agriculture. The fact that Karl König gave lectures on nutrition is not widely known. Already in the 1920s he worked together with Rudolf Hauschka and Eugen Kolisko on the topic of nutrition. König felt the need to use the lens of anthroposophy to tackle questions of nutrition.

The lectures in Prague

After leaving Silesia, König spent several months in Prague, where he gave a course for physicians and teachers. These are the four Prague lectures, which shed light on some fundamental questions of nutrition and also contain many practical indications. In the first lecture the process of nutrition is dealt with as a central and important process:

> A person who cooks ... has the task to really and honestly love what they are doing; the food then becomes imbued with love. This will influence the digestive process both in the stomach and beyond.

Secretion is, according to König, 'the rain that falls down on the digestive organs'. To have an appetite means that the secretory processes are in flow. He is keen to emphasise *how* we eat and how the human being comprising nerve-sense system, rhythmic system and metabolic-limb system relates to the threefold plant. By means of the concept of the constituent physical-soul-spiritual members of the human being, König develops a comprehensive imagination: he is not content merely to draw simple connections, but in his threefold conception König develops immense differentiation. For example in the second Prague lecture, he does not merely represent the fruits as stimulating the metabolic and limb system, but he develops a differentiated picture of the fruits themselves:

> Fruits with hard stones ... in particular ... act on the upper organisation of our blood. Pomaceous fruits such as apples and pears, with their harmonious structure, affect the middle system, while berries relate to the lower part of the organism. In berries the stones or pips have been completely dissolved and the flesh predominates.

He is not only concerned with the question of meat or vegetarian diets, as the title of the second lecture might suggest, but as with the fruits, different foodstuffs are again considered in a very differentiated way in their effect on the human organism. Even meat is subjected to König's imaginative way of looking at things, when for example he compares the digestibility of the meat of flying birds with that of goose or turkey:

> This enables us to understand why bird meat is more digestible than beef and why the meat of a domestic goose, which is land-bound, is harder to digest than pigeon meat.

In the third Prague lecture addressing the nutrition of children and babies, König even sketches a differentiated picture of sugar:

- from roots: beet sugar acts on the nerve-sense system
- from stems and leaves: cane sugar acts on the rhythmic system
- from fruits: fruit sugar (fructose) acts on the metabolic-limb system

If in this context Karl König is describing carrots as having a too strongly incarnating effect on babies, he is appealing to our differentiated observation. He is very much taking account of the relationship of forces and the subtle effects of the constituent substances of the different foodstuffs. He follows this by considering individual differences so that we should not misunderstand what he is trying to convey:

> The soul being [of the child] arrives in the realm of
> earth, of gravity; it experiences its first encounter with
> death, with the hardness of substances. This should
> not come as a shock but should take place as gently
> and lovingly as possible. For this reason a child's first
> supplementary food should be fruit, moving on to
> flower, leaf and root vegetables, in that order.

Differentiation and individualisation is expressed already in the very path of incarnation. The way in which a child announces itself and even the circumstances of its birth are signs of an individual signature and the manifestation of the destiny of a particular human being. This needs to be recognised and followed through right into the process of nutrition. Karl König is committed above all to individualised observation, free of any dogmatism. He even gives detailed consideration to the nutritional requirements of people with different temperaments.

Achieving appropriate nutrition is one of the most essential tasks of existence for König; the human being partakes in nature in a very real way through the fact that plant, mineral and animal substances are taken in, and completely transformed internally.

33

In turn human beings re-create themselves completely with the help of nature by way of sensory activity. The insertion of the phrase 'by way of sensory activity' or 'through sensory activity' points to an aspect which König – on the basis of indications by Steiner – stresses time and again in his lectures, sometimes in an apparently contradictory way. He dismisses the view that food merely serves to 'stoke the furnace', that it merely supplies energy. Man has to be seen as a physical-soul-spiritual being. Eating is a perpetual poisoning process, which is gradually overcome through the work of our digestive organs. In a graphic and pictorial way König conveys, for example, the difference between medicines and foodstuffs. Foodstuffs have to be destroyed completely and transformed, while a medicines must not be transformed. Spices occupy a transitional position between the two. This fourth lecture in Prague includes practical examples.

The breakdown of food and building up of individualised substance

König attached great importance to keeping up to date with the latest findings of scientific research. He followed current research projects with the greatest interest, and also expected his co-workers not only to share this interest, but to keep up to date on their own initiative – which was asking quite a lot. A central question for our current topic and which is still a riddle to contemporary science is the threshold nature of the *intestinal wall*. This refers to the point at which all earthly nourishment, having been processed by all the diverse digestive juices and broken down into its smallest components, is taken up by the body. How does this take place? What is it that is actually traversing the intestinal wall? In 1936 (in his first Prague lecture) and also in 1943 (in his second lecture at Heathcot) König describes the intestinal wall as impermeable and that the villi by nature tend to give off substance (like a calf suckling on the udder of a cow), while in his lectures at the agricultural conference in Thornbury in 1953, ten years later, König says the following:

Now consider the mineralised chyme substance.[1] There is no doubt that a certain amount of chyme – of this mineralised milk, this universalised substance – is now taken up through all the millions of villi of the small intestines, and carried into the lymph-capillaries which surround the intestines ...

As soon as the villi have been permeated by mineralised chyme, and the lymph vessels have taken it up, it is led upwards through the thoracic tract ... It carries the chyme up into a special vein, whence it flows into the heart. From the heart it goes upwards into our pulmonary system, where it receives through the rhythmic system the enlivening qualities of oxygen. In this way the physical chyme is lifted into the realm of living substance.

He goes on to describe how this takes place with the involvement of different organ systems and our constituent physical, soul and spiritual 'bodies'.

The process of resorption is described by science as the process by which nutrients are taken up from the stomach and intestinal tract into the blood and lymph vessels, and in an extended sense also the absorption of substances through the skin, mucous membranes or lungs. In 1958, in Botton Village in Yorkshire, in the lectures about the meteorological organs König also pointed to the possibility of 'persorption' (the non re-absorbing ingestion of microparticles in the intestinal wall):

Regarding the transit of substances through the intestinal wall, various statements have been made. Experiments in humans using radioactive markers such as a 'harmless' carbon isotope, have been used. These elements subsequently show up in different organs. The persorption rate of various toxic substances, such as DDT, is also known. This rate is even higher in infants than in adults.

35

Some of his statements may initially appear to us as somewhat absolute. I tend to attribute this rather to König's choleric temperament, as he later sometimes relativises or explains his earlier statements (for instance, resorbtion of nutrients through the intestinal wall). Here in a small circle of people he knew well, it was also simply the lively and engaged style of his lecturing. When revising something for publication himself, this immediacy and the particular choleric quality of his manner of delivery, lively and spiced with a good deal of humour, which audiences found so inspiring, was usually altered. We have left most of this directness in the texts in order to convey something of his engaged speaking.

We can also detect how König developed his knowledge and insights in the course of the years and again opened up for discussion certain topics from a wider perspective. He recalled his own attitude and enthusiasm from the twenties and thirties at the agricultural conference in Thornbury, and how he himself and all the others at the time (he was probably referring to the participating doctors and farmers) 'thought that we only needed to look around the corner, and these problems [the threefold nature of the human being, the earthly and cosmic streams of nutrition, the fallacy of motor nerves, etc.] ... would easily be solved. We were too confident, and because of this overconfidence the problems were not tackled at a deep enough level.'

In 1954, during a lecture tour of Germany, König made the following entry in his diary concerning the stream of cosmic nutrition:

> I recognise that digestion is a reversed embryonic process that leads from the particularity of the individual foodstuffs to the generality of chyme and chyle.[2] As a result chyme appears as milk and chyle as germ. This germ is 'fertilised' through the stream of cosmic nutrition. Through this fertilisation process the substance, through which the human body is perpetually renewed, is formed.

In the third Prague lecture about infant nutrition König refers to Paracelsus who described mother's milk as 'a supersensible being' ('the good mummy'), which is having a conversation with the soul being of the child, trying to coax it down to earth.

The current relevance of König's approach

The topic of König's second lecture in Prague, 'Meat or Vegetarian Food' is of particular relevance currently. Since the 1980s nutrition-dependent diseases have increasingly been the subject of nutritional research, and it is recognised that high meat consumption, as practised in first world countries, is not condu- cive to health. Currently there are various academic and govern- ment studies being undertaken in Germany to study the effects of vegetarianism. The whole subject becomes even more topical in the age of globalisation, when more and more people are com- ing to the realisation that the future of humanity cannot lie in ever-increasing meat consumption, and that over-consumption of foods rich in proteins and fats as well as sugary foods leads to symptoms of malnutrition, such as diabetes, gout, arteriosclerosis and heart disease; on the other hand, despite all developmental aid and technical improvements, world hunger is not decreasing.

It needs to be stressed here that König was not claiming gen- eral validity for his point of view: 'In the realm of nutrition there should be no sectarianism, no universally accepted point of view, but only a true understanding of the facts.'

Recent research concerning the abdominal brain confirms the validity of König's statements about the interrelationship between the intestines and the brain ('The Relation of Intestine and Brain,' p. 351) and again bear witness to the current rele- vance of his statements, as does modern psychosomatic research, which confirms the connection between psychological well-be- ing and the uptake of nutrients.

When I read the words in the first Prague lecture, 'everything, be it leaf, flower, root, be it meat or anything else, resounds, sounds, is inwardly luminous,' I am reminded of modern research dealing with biophotons. This demonstrates how all living things, including our food plants, emit minute amounts of light which can be detected and quantified.[3]

In summary it can be stated that König's approach has today lost none of its relevance; on the contrary, it might be said that only nowadays are we in a position to understand it in its wider context. König emphasised that nutrition is a very important factor in the process of incarnation of the human being and in establishing a connection with the earth. He asked a lot of his listeners: like himself, they ought to keep abreast of the most recent findings of scientific research. He also assumed that his listeners were not only familiar with the lectures by Rudolf Steiner on which his own research was based, but that they were able to study them thoroughly and had them at their fingertips.

A unique quality of König's approach is the tremendously imaginative quality of his descriptions, the thoroughness of his research and the loving seriousness with which he linked the one with the other. We encounter knowledge, scientific curiosity, enlivened by imagination and exact observation, allied to a meditatively acquired power of conception and the capacity to describe nature phenomenologically. König combines and interweaves the topics of earth and the human being, spanning the cosmic dance of the zodiac, embryology and the situation of agriculture, and the latest findings of the nutritional research of his time. König does not set out to provide answers, but to shed light on questions at different levels. He is guided by a gift for observation and a thirst for understanding and research, and provides us with an extended perspective on many questions, enabling us ultimately to act out of insight.

This book aims to make lectures that were until now largely unknown, available to a wider public. It serves to supplement and enrich Rudolf Steiner's indications on medicine, agriculture and nutrition and is an invitation to the reader to engage with the wider context of these topics.

En route to the lectures of the agricultural course, Ehrenfried Pfeiffer asked Rudolf Steiner: 'How can it happen that the spiritual impulse, and especially the inner schooling, for which you are constantly providing stimulus and guidance, bear so little fruit? Why do the people concerned give so little evidence of spiritual experiences, in spite of all their efforts? Why, worst of all, is the will for action, for the carrying out of these spiritual impulses, so weak?' Not for nothing Rudolf Steiner's reply, given in all seriousness and to Pfeiffer's complete astonishment, was: 'This is a problem of nutrition.'[4]

Anita Pedersen studied nutritional science in Giessen, Germany and at the Rural Development Programme at Emerson College, England. She has worked in Camphill community in Scotland, Wales and Germany. She has written about curative education and about nutrition.

I

1) *Feeling response to the beginning of spring in nature*
   first leaves, grasses, dew. Healing forces.
2) *In autumn the earth was nourished by the falling seeds.*
   During winter it has transformed the seeds,
   awakening with healing forces in spring.
3) *The human being experiences a sense of inner liberation.*

II

1) *What are the differences between nutrition and healing,*
   between the eating of food and [the taking of] medicines.
   In many cases of illness nutrition is disturbed.
2) *Threefoldness of the human being*
   Head —> Internal causes of illness
   Middle [rhythmic system] —> source of healing
   Metabolism —> external causes of illness
3) *Nutrition ——> digestion*
   Breathing ——> heartbeat and blood circulation
   Sense perception ——> cognition in concepts

III

1) *The process of nutrition*
   Everything has to be demolished. The human being has to
   build up everything anew.
2) *The evaluation of foodstuffs*
   Not substances but forces
   fruit sugar beef root salt
   cane sugar
   beet sugar poultry flower and fruit sugar
3) *Spices, vitamins, fragrances*

Vortrag, 22. April 1933, Prag. (on Nutrition and Healing)

I.
1) Empfindung der frühlingshaften Natur gegenüber.
Erste Blätter, Gräser, Tau. Heilende Kräfte.
2) Die Erde wurde im Herbst ernährt mit den fallenden
Samen. Sie hat im Winter die Samen verwandelt
& erwacht heilend im Frühling.
3) Der Mensch empfindet eine innerliche Befreiung.

II.
1) Welche Unterschiede bestehen zwischen Ernährung
& Heilung, essen von Nahrung & Medikamenten.
Oft ist bei Krankheit die Ernährung gestört.
2) Dreigliederung des Menschen
Haupt → innere Krankheitsursachen   Mitte → Heilung
Stoffwechsel → äußere Krankheitsursachen
3) Nahrung ————————→ Verdauung
Atmung ————————→ Herzschlag & Blutumlauf
Wahrnehmung ————————→ Erkennen in Begriffen.

III.
1) Der Prozeß der Ernährung.
Alles muss zerschlagen werden.   Neu muss der Mensch
alles aufbauen.
2) Die Bewertung der Nahrungsmittel.
nicht Stoffe sondern Kräfte
Fruchtzucker   Rindfleisch   Wurzel   Salz
Rohrzucker
Rübenzucker   Vogelfleisch   Blüte & Frucht   Zucker
3) Gewürze, Vitamine, Duftstoffe.

*Notes by Karl König for a lecture on April 22, 1933 in Prague
about nutrition and healing. (On that day in Germany the
edict restricting the work of Jewish doctors was issued.)*

41

IV

1) Nutrition demolishes everything

2) Healing preserves/maintains everything. Medicines enter the body not in order to be transformed, but to transform.

3) Lime blossoms

Lemon balm leaves   blackthorn fruits

Gentian roots

4) Allopathy and homoeopathy

V

1) The transformation of nutritional power into healing power

2) We transform the substances to enable us to breathe properly and to develop clear understanding

3) The Last Supper

Nutrition is transformed into healing power

A Being takes the world into Himself

as a pure mirror, and that constitutes healing.

4) Even your tears turn into dew of blessing

You weep, and lo, the meadow smiles.

Illness and healing
Nutrition and healing
The illnesses of our
time in their spiritual nature
and social significance

IV.
1) Ernährung zerschlägt alles
2) Heilung erhält alles. Heilmittel gehen in den Körper nicht um verwandelt zu werden, sondern um zu verwandeln,
3) Lindenblüten
   Enzianwurzeln   Melissenblätter , Schlehdorn Frucht
4) Allopathie s Homöopathie

V.
1) Die Verwandlung von Nahrungskraft in Heilkraft.
2) Wir verwandeln die Stoffe , um richtig atmen
          u klar erkennen zu können
3) Das Abendmahl =
   Ernährung wird Heilung.
   Ein Wesen nimmt die Welt in sich
   als reiner Spiegel, das ist Heilung.
4) Auch deine Träne ward zum Segensstaue
   Du weinest sich, es lacht die Aue.

Krankheit u Heilung
Ernährung u Heilung

Die Krankheiten unseren Zeit in ihrer geistigen Bedeutung u spätere Bedeutung.

Cosmic and Earthly Nutrition

Lectures for physicians and teachers in Prague, 1936

1 Nutrition in General

Lecture 1, April 1936

Your invitation to give these lectures on nutrition has provided me with a welcome opportunity to address some essential aspects of this subject, stimulated particularly by an experience of the conditions that I have encountered here in Prague.[1]

Walking around the streets of Prague, you notice that there is a butcher's or a pastry shop on almost every street corner. This is hardly an uplifting sight, as it falls to the doctor to witness the devastating effect of poor nutrition on the physical, psychological and spiritual organisation of the human being. It is indeed a truly depressing sight. Nutrition not only affects physical aspects of life here on earth. My hope is that, if we achieve nothing else through this course, we will at least manage to establish a comprehensive perspective with regard to the subject of nutrition. We have to realise how nutrition is among the most essential aspects of existence; irrespective of whether we are ideologists or idealists, we should not undervalue those who attach importance to nutrition. This is not to say that nutrition should become the centre of all existence. We need to adopt an impartial approach to the whole matter of eating and of digestion, to the whole subject of metabolism and the uptake of nourishment if we are to reach any true understanding. Through ingesting food we really partake in nature through the fact that we take plant, mineral and animal substances into our whole organisation and then transform them completely within this organisation, building ourselves up and forming our bodies on the basis of this actual relationship to nature.

Nutrition also needs to be considered in its relation to nationality; different peoples may be identified by the character of their food.[2] Travelling for example through France, Italy, England, Germany, Austria or any other country, it becomes evident that everywhere the basic character of the people comes to expression in their nutrition; and that nutrition, in turn, exerts a strong influence on the people. Whether we eat noodles or dumplings, food affects our whole organism. For example, one feels a different person when living in England, where one is obliged to eat unfamiliar foods which often appear tasteless and bland. In Paris, by contrast, one is presented with foods which have been prepared in an unbelievably delicate and ensouled way – seven or eight individual dishes in succession. The French still have much by way of traditional knowledge and they are instinctive masters of the art of using spices for flavouring; however, their style has become rather stereotyped. One becomes a different person yet again if one lives and eats here in Prague. This is not intended as a criticism of Prague.

One can see how in each country tradition has been preserved in the style of eating and is still maintained, despite changes during the last twenty or thirty years. This has given rise to the health food movement that attempts to improve health through modifying nutrition. Among them are those who advocate eating only raw food, or only vegetarian food, those who say that one only remains healthy if one also eats meat, or that if you eat meat, you will become ill. The approaches of the different schools are quite sectarian, and I do not propose to defend a particular position or state that only this or that type of food should be eaten. Mankind as a whole is so all-encompassing that nutritional advice cannot be reduced simply to choosing between meat and raw food. Advice needs to be individualised, for example when recommending feeding schedules for babies or recipes for families. To offer such advice depends in turn on cultivating a much deeper understanding of what nutrition involves.

The saying that the way to a man's heart is through his stomach is not entirely without justification. The important thing is not that one merely learns to cook, but that one does so in a particular way. It is my experience that women have lost touch with the art of cooking. The feeling for food has been lost, not because cooking should be exclusively a task for women, but because people generally have lost the feeling for the spiritual behind the material. We no longer even distinguish plant from mineral substance, flower from leaf or root, and have no idea what the cosmic forces are that are weaving and working in them. We have lost the art of handling food in the right way. The aim is not that we should all become gourmets, but that we should gain an understanding and respect for the sacred nature of food preparation, of eating and of digesting. The greatest religious images are concealed in the depiction of 'sitting at the table'. Not only hygienic procedures but ritual traditions are found in all religions in connection with partaking in meals, be it in the Buddhist, Jewish or Christian religion. These traditions are hygienic but above all they are sacramental procedures connected with the act of 'sitting at table'.

A person who cooks also has the task to really and honestly love what they are doing; the food then becomes imbued with love. This will influence the digestive process both in the stomach and beyond.

Today I do not intend to focus on food as such, but to refer to it only by way of introducing the complex field of nutrition. If we are to speak about food, we need to speak about the individual ingredients. Today I only want to address the process of nutrition and metabolism, because the most ridiculous and erroneous views prevail in this domain.

We really do not know what takes place when we ingest foods. Science has us believe that food is nothing but the fuel for the human oven. Coal – that is, the food – is shovelled in and burnt and from this, energy is generated that feeds the organs and muscles and enables us to live. We have to eat in order to live. But if eating were really so simple, we would simply not survive and would starve. It is impossible to hold the concept that our body is constructed from the individual ingredients and particles – this is absolutely incorrect! The individual substances we take in are transformed and enter as nutritional components into our organism, become part of our lung, our liver and so forth and provide us, among other things, with the power of thinking. We need to find a comprehensive picture of this process, which takes place when we sit at table, eat, take in foods, when nature enters our organism and is transformed by us and rebuilt. We can only understand what is taking place if we consider the human being as a whole, taking into account not only the physical organisation, but evaluating the whole human being existing as physical-soul-spiritual being.

What is the most essential aspect to be considered with regard to nutrition? The process of eating food is one of permanent poisoning, and only through the activity of our digestive organs is this poisoning process gradually overcome. Consider the following experiment: imagine that milk were to be injected rather than drunk, thereby avoiding the digestive process altogether and entering the organism directly. If this were to be done, it would poison the organism and induce an immune reaction. This is why milk has even been injected to treat different illnesses, inducing a fever that in turn breaks down the milk.[3] When you drink milk, of course you don't develop a fever, because the milk is destroyed and dissolved in the process of passing through the whole digestive tract. The poisoning processes are thereby halted and we are nourished. If milk enters our body directly, bypassing this process, we are poisoned. During research on nutrients defined as 'vitamins', scientists have had to realise that nutrition is not simply a matter of individual nutrients building up and nourishing our body.

Twenty years ago it was stated that milk is a good source of nutrition. Consequently, so it was said, its individual nutrients must also be good, so people tried to feed rats and mice by giving them the individual nutrients in the same ratio as found in milk. The same fats, the same proteins and carbohydrates were taken, and these isolated substances were fed to mice. The mice fed on milk lived on happily, but those fed on the individual substances died a miserable death within a short space of time. At that time people were not yet able to differentiate between a composite physiological entity such as milk, and its broken down components. What scientists then postulated was that there must be a substance contained in the milk that had not yet been isolated, and that it needed to be found in order to understand why one group of mice died while the other continued to live. The result was the birth of a new branch of science – the science of vitamins. A vast variety of substances was found, but to manufacture vitamin substances will not be straightforward, because with vitamins we are not dealing primarily with isolated substances, but with interconnected forces.[4] Nowadays scientists recognise that it is not only the substances that nourish us, but that something else is required, namely forces. The nature of these forces will be described later.

As we are aiming to develop a comprehensive understanding of the subject of nutrition, the essential relationship of the human being to the environment needs to be taken into our consideration. In the case of the human head this relationship is differentiated in a threefold way, expressing itself in:

- The forehead: this is connected with what is conveyed to us by our senses – light, sound, etc.
- The nose: this is connected with everything to do with respiration.
- The mouth: this is connected with what enters our organism through nutrition.

Let us take a closer look at these three levels of the relationship between the human being and the outer world, as they manifest through the senses, through breathing and through nutrition. The whole sensory process takes place above, in the region of the head; the breathing process takes place in the middle system – the system of lung and heart – and the whole process of nutrition takes place lower down, in the activity of limbs and metabolism. It is possible to understand the human being as a threefold being simply through the fact that we look at these three complexes through the five senses of the head, through the breathing and through nutrition.

If we study the breathing process, it becomes evident in the first instance that this relationship does not consist merely of intake, but that it also manifests a counter-thrust. We do not only breathe in but we also breathe out. This constitutes the entire rhythmic system, which permeates our existence from birth to death. Breathing in – breathing out, breathing in – breathing out, etc.

In the case of the sensory and nutrition processes we are aware of only one side of the processes; the counterpart is unknown. We assimilate the images, we form concepts and pictures. The environment streams in through the senses, but what is it that streams back? In nutrition we take in the substances, we breathe them in, as it were, but what is it that streams back? Only when we come to know what it is that actually streams back into us as a counter-thrust to the uptake of food, when we also understand the breathing-out process of nutrition, will we gain a comprehensive understanding of nutrition as a whole.

In answer to the questions you posed,[5] I am proposing that nutrition needs to be understood not only in terms of the intake of substances, but in the context of these, the three levels of the human being's connection with his environment. The breathing in of the world and the breathing out of something of ourselves: this wonderful exchange with the world. The human being takes up oxygen and gives out carbon dioxide, takes up various substances from the air and in turn gives off others. Even when we consider the sensory aspects – light, sound, smell, taste – there is not only the stream of taking in, but also the counter-stream. Sense activity is not only taking in, but also giving out. The eye does not only take light from the sun, but also gives out light to the environment, and the ear gives out sound to the environment.

In the works of Plato, for example, who still had knowledge of the ancient mysteries, we find an awareness that sensory activity in particular entails not only a comprehensive taking-in of substances but also a 'breathing out' process. He knew how the human being is simultaneously thrusting outwards, sounding through the ear, and in that way engaging with the environment. Goethe said that the eye has been created out of the light, in conjunction with the light and for the light – he described it as really sunlike, as having an inner radiance. We find this principle – only 'pulled down' in a physical sense – when we study the different animals: cats and other predators, for example, produce certain substances that emanate light which one can actually see. The light that human beings also radiate, we are not able to see, nor can we hear the sound; yet it exists. Here too a breathing-out process in relation to the breathing-in process is taking place.

Let us now consider how the breathing-out aspect of the nutrition process may be understood.

We don't only consume food, but we also emanate a certain counter-stream into the world when we eat. Where is this to be found? The fact that today I and others are able even to raise this question is due to the fact that Dr Steiner has provided extremely vital insights out of anthroposophy that are capable of shedding light on this whole subject. I would like to describe what has come to light in the most recent scientific research as a basis for then discovering together with you the counter-stream, enabling us thereby to gain a more comprehensive understanding of nutrition.

Some thirty years ago a Russian physiologist, Ivan Pavlov, performed some nutritional experiments that produced some curious and unique results, but which could not be made use of because people did not understand their practical relevance. He showed that when we take in food, it is enveloped in saliva in the mouth, arrives in the stomach, which gives off its own secretions, as do the gall bladder, the liver, the intestines, etc. In brief, in the whole of the digestive tract substances are flowing, enveloping and destroying what has been taken in. The moment food is taken in, via the mouth, the oesophagus (food pipe), the stomach, the intestines, it is as if rain had started falling inside our organism; it is a marvellous and incredible rain that falls on everything that has been ingested. Pavlov wanted to investigate how it rains. He used dogs in his experiments. I do not wish to express any ethical judgment about this, but am only concerned with reporting the results. Pavlov surgically transected the oesophagi of dogs and then sewed them together so that what had been eaten would flow out again at the back. The following could then be observed: The moment the food has been taken in through the mouth, not only does salivary secretion begin, but the whole stomach and intestinal tract begins to 'rain'. It is clear that the gastric secretions do not only originate in the stomach or the intestinal secretions in the intestines, but that the moment food has been taken in, incredible processes of secretion begin, throughout the whole digestive tract.

Pavlov was very inventive. He then placed a cat in front of the dog; the dog became angry, and with the onset of anger the stomach and intestinal secretion ceased. Everything came to a standstill; the dog no longer digested anything. It is important to realise that through a psychological shock everything can seize up, since this also applies to the human being: anger can make eating impossible; afterwards hunger returns. This experiment also relates to human nature in general: rage, anger and fright prevent the flow of secretions, and this inhibits nutrition. Pavlov demonstrated something else: Being a skilled surgeon, he opened up the stomach of a dog and stitched it to the skin, so that he could insert food directly into the stomach through a hole. He was able to insert bread, meat, dog biscuits, etc. into the stomach. As the dog was not aware that anything had entered his stomach, everything remained there unchanged. It might as well have been stones. There was not a drop of secretion. How can this be accounted for? Pavlov also conditioned dogs by sounding a certain trumpet note whenever the dogs were given food. Then he would no longer give food, but only sound the trumpet. At that very moment saliva, gastric and intestinal juices began to flow, indicating that the flow of the digestive juices is not dependent on the presence of physical food, but on the psychological response.

We know that when we see appetising food it is literally mouth-watering: the mouth actually begins to water. It is the psychological impact of the food that causes the saliva to flow; on the other hand, we may sit at an ever so richly laden table without experiencing any appetite. To experience appetite is tantamount to the flow of digestive juices. This flow is dependent on the psychological condition of the person or animal. To a large degree nutrition depends not so much on *what* we eat but *how* we eat. This is easily said, but much harder to implement and even harder to understand. In the olden days people did not, as we do today, rush into any old eating house, eat something while standing, and move on; people took their meals rhythmically, they sat at table, said a grace together and then started the meal together. This attitude was not just a matter of social convention – in those days food preparation and eating were still experienced as sacred processes, and I doubt whether there were as many metabolic or intestinal disorders then as there are today.

The important consideration is not so much *what* one eats but *how* one eats, a significant number of illnesses could be prevented if we could only learn once again to eat in the right way and bring appropriate understanding to the digestive processes. Nowadays people don't want to spend their time in this way, but they lose far more time in the long run if they have to consult the doctor as a result of the habit of eating in haste, oblivious of the consequences. We are then no longer able to perceive what we eat; we lose our ability to taste what is sweet, what is sour or bitter or salty. Moreover, we do not fully grasp that in reality we partake of a particular cosmic force when we experience a bitter taste, a different one when we taste something sour or something sweet; we are no longer aware of this relationship. Who is aware nowadays that the whole flowering and fruiting process in the plant is connected with sugar, whereas the root process is connected with the tart and salty? What factors are essentially connected with the tart and with the sour taste? Nowadays it does not occur to people that cosmic forces might be able to come to our consciousness while eating. This completely passes people by through the haste of daily life and through the abstract element in their lives – we no longer taste what is being revealed through the taste!

To become conscious in this tasting process would be an essential task in learning to eat, one which could begin by taking the trouble to sit round the table in a mood of calm, saying a grace that is in keeping with present-day consciousness and really focussing on what is taking place when, through partaking in nourishment, cosmic forces enter our organism. Then eating could begin by starting to sense what is bitter, salt, sour – anything belonging to the food that generates taste. After the food enters the mouth, ensalivation immediately follows. This in itself constitutes a marvellous process that varies considerably, depending on whether we are eating meat, vegetables or bread. It is a vital fact that saliva is constituted quite differently, depending on the nature of what has been taken in. But how does this differentiation actually come about, depending on the food taken in? How does the salivary gland know how much to produce? We have three salivary glands.[6] They are constituted in such a way that one of them produces a saltier, the next one a more basic and the third one a more acidic secretion, in this way giving rise to a differentiation. If we eat meat, the character of secretion is a completely different from when we are eating bread.

A fundamental question we need to ask if we hope to understand the question of nutrition, is how this difference in the saliva can be accounted for. The question we could ask is, can the salivary glands think? For it is only out of the sphere of thinking that your secretions can be so precisely co-ordinated that they are able to exert the right influence on the food that has been taken in. Perhaps these salivary glands are indeed able to think! In any event, they not only secrete, but to do so in a *rational* manner: This implies that they are not only glands but also sense organs. Every gland in our body is only secondarily a gland; for the major part of its existence it is a sense organ. These three salivary glands in the mouth and throat region that produce their secretions in response to the food taken in are only able to perform this task with such precision because they also incorporate a sensory function in relation to the ingested food. Thanks to this sense perception – and this is quite distinct from the nerves – they, as it were, hear the sound, the inner word of the food taken in. For everything, be it leaf, flower, root, be it meat or anything else, resounds, sounds, is inwardly luminous; our salivary glands perceive this, and based on this perception are able to respond by giving out their secretions.

Then the food passes through the cavity of the mouth and enters the oesophagus. Carbohydrates already begin to be broken down in the oral cavity, and when they have reached the stomach, another substance is added. The secretions added in the stomach are not only aimed at the destruction of the carbohydrates, but also of the proteins, both of plant and animal origin. But in the stomach the same process is found as in the mouth: the stomach secretions are constituted completely differently, depending on the type of plant, flower, root; the quantities of salts, acids, pepsin, etc., are different, because even in the stomach the food constituents are still able to radiate, to sound; the glands then look and listen. Out of this interplay of radiance, seeing, sounding and listening, the right enzymes are secreted.

These continue the process of destroying the food or, as it were, detoxifying it. Food does not remain a foreign body when taken in. Cabbage does not remain cabbage after we have eaten it, nor when the wolf eats a lamb does it become a lamb. Cabbage and kale are rendered non-toxic, destroyed as distinct entities; milk is destroyed, meat is destroyed as an entity and dissolved into its constituent parts through the fact that the resounding and the radiance begins in the glands and that they respond by secreting these digestive juices. If someone has a gastric dysfunction, it is not necessarily due to eating the wrong foods, but because the wrong gastric juice has been secreted due to a disturbance in the sensory process.

There are gastric illnesses in which the person gives off the same gastric juices for meat, vegetables and other foods, and as a result the food is inadequately broken down. It is not the secretory process but the sensory process that is disturbed. The stomach is not a sack, as people think, but an incredibly complex entity that lives inside us. If this entity loses its capacity for hearing and seeing the food, it becomes like a blind or a deaf man stumbling along. He will then not know his way about, and he will have something lying inside him that he is not able to deal with. This manifests as some form of stomach upset, or perhaps as gastroenteritis.

Let us follow the further progress of the digestive process:

- in the mouth carbohydrates are already digested, then
- in the stomach the proteins are broken down and
- in the small intestine the fatty substances.

These three stages of digestion will play a significant role in our future deliberations.

There is nothing arbitrary in the fact that we first digest carbohydrates, then proteins and finally fats. It is in fact a stepwise progression leading from carbohydrates via proteins to fats. When the fats themselves have been digested, the remaining food has turned into chyle, a homogeneous pulp found in the small intestine. And now a difficult chapter begins. Endless effort and much diligence have been expended on thousands of experiments designed to investigate what happens to this chyle in the small intestine. To this day science has to admit that it knows next to nothing about the way the dissolved, digested substances of foods pass from the intestine into the bloodstream. It is a difficult question. All around the intestinal wall are the lymph vessels which merge into the blood vessels. The belief is that the chyle passes through the intestinal wall, building up the lymph and the blood. If we investigate this, we find tiny fat droplets which may be connected with the fats that have been digested; there are no, or only minimal quantities of, proteins and no traces of carbohydrates.[7]

Thus we have:

Carbohydrates	none
Proteins	some
Fats	quite a lot

What has become of all these substances? This intestinal wall is a real barrier, and if we do not take seriously the fact that no chyle can pass through this barrier, we will fail to understand what happens with our food and our nutrition. To put it bluntly, it is materialistic nonsense to believe that foods pass through the intestinal wall; what remains inside will eventually be excreted as stools. But only the minutest amount will traverse this wall. We have to be clear about the fact that the intestinal wall constitutes a substantial barrier; if we study it, we find that it consists of a system made up of a multitude of extremely tiny and fine microvilli. It is believed that they break up the food substances and absorb them. Now villi exist everywhere in nature, not in order to absorb but to excrete. Consider, for instance, the udder of a cow. The calf does not attach itself to it in order for the udder to receive something from the calf, but the other way round. Were the former to be the case, the calf itself would be the source of nutrient substance in relation to the cow! Now try to imagine a calf sucking on the intestinal villi, sucking out the intestinal secretions just as the calf is sucking the milk from the udder. Nutrients do not in reality penetrate to the other side of the intestinal wall. The process of nutrition takes place up to this point, beyond which the actual metabolic process begins. Nutrition and metabolism are in fact two completely different processes. In order to understand metabolism we need to adopt a different point of departure.

In recent decades people have struggled to explain the phenomenon that some seemingly quite dull animals have quite complicated brains, while other animals – as well as human beings – which are very clever have less complicated brains. The dolphin, which has the most complicated brain, is not after all characterised by any flashes of genius. Then scientists stumbled upon a remarkable phenomenon: those animals that have the most brain convolutions also have the most intestinal convolutions. It was then suggested that the two phenomena are somehow connected. It was discovered that there is a close relationship between brain and intestine both in animals and in humans.[8] Only those animals which have a large intestine also tend to develop a cerebrum; moreover, there is not a single animal with a large intestine that does not have a cerebrum. This does not mean that the animal develops a cerebrum because there is a large intestine, but that there is a parallel development, in which the cerebrum does not arise first, but where both arise together.

We need to consider the significance of this. Neither in animals nor in the human being is Paul Julius Möbius' statement true, that women are less intelligent because they have smaller brains than men.[9] Because the brain of a woman is 200 to 300 grams lighter than that of a man, he speaks of physiological feeble-mindedness. However, both in the animal kingdom and in the human being it is evident that these things are indeed closely connected with intestinal development.

Some strange characters are to be found in the world of science. About twenty years ago – at the same time as Möbius wrote the above statement – the significant researcher Metchnikov made out a case for removing the large intestines in humans, solely because it did not apparently serve any useful purpose.[10] In fact each part has its function in the overall human organism, and this would then have been destroyed. I mention this because in America they started removing all appendices from infants, as they did not consider they had any purpose and only caused inflammations. The experiment failed, as most of these poor children died a year or so later. An inflamed appendix corresponds to a sore throat in the abdomen, but the appendix is as necessary as the tonsils are in the throat.

We will only be able to understand the connection between the brain and the development of the intestines if we look for the counter-processes to nutrition. We have learnt that nutrition does not depend only on the foods. Pavlov's experiments have shown that nutrition has a close connection with psychological factors – how we relate to life, whether we are joyful, sad or melancholic by nature. The flow of the secretions is based much more on a psychological than on a physical process. The food needs to be dissolved and destroyed within the whole gastro-intestinal tract of mouth, stomach and intestine, and then the residue or pulp encounters the intestinal wall and cannot proceed any further.

Another significant experiment has come to light in recent times, which was not carried out at universities, but in seclusion. This is the experience of Therese of Konnersreuth.[11] I do not wish to speak about her visions, which would be a task in its own right, but only about the fact that this woman was evidently able to survive without food for many years, and that to this day, whether we like it or not, not the least bit of understanding has been forthcoming to explain how it is possible to live without food. She lived under the supervision of doctors, church ministers and her father. The doctors kept her under surveillance for many years; she did not take in any food, apart from receiving the host once a week in church. I do not propose to pass judgment about the reliability or otherwise of her intuitions. As a doctor it is rather my responsibility to contemplate such an experiment involving the relationship between nature and this human being, who did indeed live for many years without food and was still able to exist. This example has nothing to do with the practice of going on hunger strike as a stunt or for some other reason. I consider it important to develop a proper appreciation of this. It is seemingly a fact that a human being can live for years without taking in food, even maintaining normal bodily excretions without ingesting anything. What does this signify?

The entire cerebral system is connected with the intestinal organisation; just as our brain in its structure is anatomically connected with the intestines, so the whole metabolic process of our intestines is connected with a supersensible process, which takes place through the brain, through the senses. Regarding nutrition, Steiner pointed out that we should not just look at the physical stream of nutrition that enters our organism, but at a second stream, the *cosmic stream of nutrition*.[12] This cosmic nutrition stream is one which, unlike the normal nutrition stream, does not enter our organism via mouth, stomach, intestine, but is the counter-stream to the physical nutrition stream. It enters our organism through the senses, through the brain. We do not only perceive the light as colour, not only tone as sound, but with light and sound and all the other sense impressions, cosmic substance enters our organism, and we assimilate this into our body. The secretions I have called 'rain', are fundamentally nothing other than the raining down of the cosmic nutrition stream. When food impacts psychologically via sense perception, this cosmic nutrition stream begins to flow, and we see this in the streaming of the digestive secretions in the saliva, in stomach and intestines. There the whole stream of cosmic nutrition pours into us through the sense organs and subsequently via the brain. We are linked to a nutrition process not just through the intake of food but also through light and sound.

Dr Steiner went so far as to state that spiritually informed study of the whole digestive and metabolic process would reveal that there is only one substance in our organism which is built up out of physical foods, namely the grey matter of the brain; everything else is built up out of these cosmic processes. Fundamentally, physical nutrition is required in order to stimulate the flow of the cosmic nutrition stream in the right way. Nutrition itself is necessary for this reason – something that Therese of Konnersreuth was able to accomplish out of her peculiar constitution by means of the communion host, which she received once a week. And the nature of different kinds of food, whether it be flower, leaf, root or whatever, stimulate the cosmic streams each in their particular way. The ingested substances essentially come to a halt at the intestinal wall; only the final remnants pass over into the lymph. The pulp has turned into a chaos, just as happens in the fertilised ovum. Thus human beings only acquire their form through the fact that the soul penetrates the organs, bringing the supersensible into contact with what remains as physical substance after its form has been completely annihilated. The chaotic substances of the chyle then enter the lymph. In this way the entire configuration of the cosmic stream is taken in and builds up the whole human being.

We have to accompany the path of nutrition in our mind up to the intestinal wall and then appreciate the outcome, namely chaotic substance. Then, in response to its passing through the barrier, the cosmic stream takes hold of it and builds it up into the new physical human being.

This cosmic nutrition stream penetrates the body in the process of descending from the supersensible, building up the physical substances that are found in liver, lung, bones, muscles – that is, throughout the whole organism. And the final remnants of fats and proteins that pass into the lymph, rise upwards with the blood and are deposited in the brain. This is the most material and physical substance we have in our body. The grey cerebral cortex is actually built up out of material substance, while everything else is built up by the cosmic nutrition stream. Perhaps this idea may enable us to understand a phenomenon that we often find puzzling: the fact that some people are quite thin; although they eat a lot they don't put on weight, while others are rather fat; they eat little, and yet put on weight. Perhaps we may be able to appreciate the reason for this if we know that we put on weight through the cosmic nutrition stream, depending on whether it flows in a good or a bad way. Therefore there is no merit in being either fat or thin, even though it relates to cosmic forces. Dr Steiner called the fat of pigs a cosmic fat because it is not derived from the food.[13] We too do not carry earthly but cosmic fat on our bodies, and yet we have no reason to be proud of it. In any case, bodily substance does not derive from the physical but from the cosmic realm. It derives from that nutrition stream which comes down from the supersensible realm; just as this supersensible stream becomes physical, the physical substances become supersensible. Whatever substance is destroyed or annihilated, nothing is actually lost; everything is transformed and becomes supersensible substance, just as the supersensible substance from the cosmic realm becomes sense-perceptible.

What we have now discerned is the breathing process in the sphere of nutrition: substance is breathed in and passed over into the supersensible realm. The supersensible stream, which becomes physical by means of the brain and the sense organs, is turned into physical substance while the physical stream is transferred to the supersensible realm. If we contemplate these two streams, we come to understand what it means to eat and to say grace before a meal. This is what Angelus Silesius formulated on the basis of the gospels:[14]

> It is not the bread that feed us; what feeds us in the bread
> Is God's eternal word, is spirit and is life.

We can take these words quite literally. It really isn't the bread, but it is the light and the life of the whole world that enter our organism through the cosmic nutrition stream. We can become bearers of this cosmic stream through the fact that we take in physical nourishment. We are dealing with radiant cosmic nourishment and the ingestion of physical bread. From this perspective it becomes clear that it is preferable, even essential that we don't eat meals in a rush without due regard for what it involves; why it is important to regard nutrition as one of the most spiritual of all actions we perform in life and not just as a material necessity or indulgence. I have tried, by way of introduction, to present the full scope of the subject under consideration.

2 Vegetarian Food or Meat?

Lecture 2, April 1936

In my previous lecture I addressed the most fundamental aspects of the processes underlying nutrition and how these encompass every aspect of the human organisation – how in the nutrition process we are not only dealing with the process that we can describe scientifically, and which we can know and study in every detail; that is, the ingestion of the individual foods through the mouth, the oesophagus, the stomach and the intestinal tract; the annihilation, the breaking down of all meat, plant and mineral substances into the separate constituents of the food. If we merely consider this single stream that runs from the outer world into the inner world through the mouth and the whole stomach and intestinal tract, we will not gain a comprehensive understanding of nutrition in its totality. To do so, we need to make at a comparison with the breathing process, in which it is obvious that not only is the process of breathing-in involved, but also that of breathing-out. We have to contemplate the breathing-out process and realise that it is equally important to discern the *counter-process* to physical nutrition amidst the various observations we have been able to make.

What was described as the cosmic nutrition stream revealed itself. And we were able to show how this comes to expression in our organism in what streams as the rain of the digestive juices inside the mouth, the stomach and the intestines; how this stream of rain pours down upon the food when we eat, or even in response to food-related stimuli, hunger or psychological events connected with the intake of food. This rainfall of the digestive juices is a sign that the cosmic nutrition stream is flowing; it flows into the human organisation and from it builds up everything that eventually becomes the physical substance of our bodies. And we encountered the remarkable statement by Rudolf Steiner, that our whole organism is not built up out of what we eat – through the physical nutrition stream – but that fundamentally our whole organism – bones, muscles, nerves – in its substance is built up out of forces deriving from the cosmic nutrition stream. According to Steiner, only the grey cerebral cortex in the head is built up out of the physical nutrients.[1]

Our task is to develop a clear picture of what takes place on the other side of the intestinal wall when the individual foods have really been broken down, to ask ourselves what happens with these individual substances that have reached an end point, have been separated out into their constituent elements, into relatively simple compounds of carbon dioxide, oxygen, hydrogen sulphide, perhaps even sulphur. In the previous lecture I presented a picture as an indication of what our organism does with the broken-down, disintegrated substances when the cosmic nutrition streams enter in. By analogy, when in a human being or an animal the act of fertilisation has reduced the substance within the fertilised ovum to a chaotic state, the fact that an embryonic animal or human form then arises, is not of primary importance. Rather, we must grasp the picture that it is the soul of the incarnating human being, the spirit streaming down that binds and sculpts this disintegrated chaotic substance. All food substance that is transferred into the bloodstream from the chyle represents just such chaos.[2] And the cosmic nutrition stream is none other than the spirit that streams down and assembles these chaotic food substances into completely human substance. In this context, it is not possible to give more than brief indications to this effect.

We have four principal organs in our body, both sense-perceptible and supersensible, which act as four guardians or gateways in relation to these internal substance streams. It is through these particular organs that the cosmic stream is guided so that it takes up this chaotic substance and forms it under human influence. These are heart, lung, liver and kidney. They have a much more significant task than is apparent to a superficial view. For example, it is not the most important task of the lung to conduct the stream of air into the organism, or of the kidney to excrete urine, or the liver to produce bile; these organs have a far broader, more comprehensive task within the whole ecological system of our organism.

In the previous lecture reference was made to the salivary gland and the other glands that give off secretions in response to sensory stimuli. They can therefore be regarded as sense organs, which receive not the physical but the cosmic stream. Depending on how they receive it, they 'alchemically' engender the whole human being. It is important to consider lung, liver, kidney and heart, and observe these organs more closely. These four organs are connected with the four archetypal forces of the realm of life: earth, air, water and fire, referred to by the alchemists as the four elements. They live and weave in these archetypal cosmic forces, forming, permeating and building up the bodily organism. This picture requires further explanation, but can only be outlined here.

Earth is connected with all the characteristic tendencies expressed by the lung, *water* with the function of the liver, *air* with the activity of the kidney, and *fire* weaves and lives in our heart.[3] Just as these four organs interact, they link together earth, water, air and fire, forming the human organisation out of the cosmic organisation. This image is intended to provide a coherent picture of what was said in the previous lecture, and which is now to be elaborated. In order to penetrate into the nutrition processes, we need to look not only at the human being but at the kingdoms of nature that supply this nutrition: the animals, plants and minerals. Science tends not to pay much attention to this aspect. It refers to proteins, carbohydrates, fats, mineral nutrients and vitamins. From a certain point of view such an approach is justified. It is important to know how much of which substance is contained in the individual foodstuffs. However, this approach is not a comprehensive one. We need to go further and should not settle for the position of the modern nutritional physiologist and pathologist, who write in the introduction to a book on dietetics that since we obtain our food from plant sources as well as from the animal world, in the first instance it is theoretically immaterial from where we obtain our foodstuffs, as the body encompasses them in a species-specific way, adapting them to the nature of its own organism.

This approach is a quantitative one, and its influence extends right into social life. In London and New York, restaurants provide menu cards that list the calorific value of every dish. People sit down and work out how much they should be eating, and make their choice of dishes accordingly. (How the food tastes, prepared entirely according these strict criteria, and what it looks like, is particularly evident in England.) The quantitative approach that ignores the plant or animal origin of the protein, saying: protein is protein, carbohydrates are carbohydrates, fats are fats, does not address the most important issues. We will now try to transcend this approach and pursue a qualitative direction when considering individual foods.

There is, in fact, a growing trend to study quality, to consider the whole human being rather than to analyse everything into its constituent parts and to measure them. However, real insight is necessary to be able to represent this trend effectively and to develop a convincing qualitative approach to nutrition. It is not a matter of indifference whether we consume protein in the form of a piece of veal or in the form of a potato, or carbohydrates in the form of a potato or in the form of bread. It is possible to verify this by means of a simple experiment. We may eat a large quantity of bread, and the following day eat a similar quantity of potatoes. We will notice that a lot of bread causes the abdomen to bloat. Eating a lot of potatoes causes our consciousness to become dull during the process of digestion. Having eaten too many potatoes, we may have difficulty writing an important letter, doing a calculation or thinking something through. One feels heavy and experiences the need to lie down. What is the cause of this?

The carbohydrates and starches in potatoes and those in bread are chemically not that different; however, there are two fundamental differences in the substance, in the natural context associated with the potato and the bread. However absurd what I am about to say may appear at first, we digest bread with our intestine and with the four glands, the liver, heart, lung and kidney, but we digest the potato with a completely different organ, namely our midbrain.[4] We are only able to understand this if we take a qualitative view of the individual foodstuffs. This is immaterial when we take the simple view that carbohydrates are carbohydrates, but it is important to understand how one or the other nutritional substance affects the human being. We will only be able to understand this if we can really perceive human beings in the context of their relationship to the processes of nature. Whether we eat meat, plant or mineral food makes a big difference, because plants, animals and minerals simply have completely different affinities and relationships with the different members of the human organisation.

We may say: here we have the minerals, and above them the plants, and still higher the animals. It would be wrong to place human beings still higher, as they encompass everything. But when we take in the first, second, third levels of substance from the realm of nature, we take in developmental stages of the cosmos. When we eat plants they don't stimulate the same members of our organism as do foods of animal origin. Plants possess comprehensive faculties within the natural world; they are able to build up the highest substances out of individual lower substances. You know that plants are able to synthesise carbohydrates – and several other high grade substances which are in our organism – simply from carbon dioxide, and link it with the sunlight by means of chlorophyll, the green substance found in plants.

Thus mineral substances, which are lower, are taken up by the plants – and these in turn are taken up by animals; therefore, when we look at the plant, we have in front of us a transformed and elevated mineral realm, and in the animal an elevated and transformed plant realm. So, if as a human being we eat the plant, we have as it were to transform it first into an animal, and from the animal into a human. But when we eat food derived from animals, we don't have to traverse this double route in our digestion and nutrition; we simply transform it into human substance. On the other hand we have to transform mineral food into the plant, animal and human realm; that is, when we take in minerals as food, we ourselves actually have to carry out all the stages of transformation.

- Mineral into plant, animal and human substance
- Plant into animal and human substance
- Animal into human substance

Now, on the basis of this picture, one might think that the simplest thing would be to eat meat as this means we would have to do the least amount of work. However, this is not the case. Looking at people who eat a lot of meat, we may notice that they have a certain excess or surplus in their bodily organisation, manifesting as depository conditions and a deficit in their soul organisation with respect to mental alertness and concentration. This is due to the fact that the inner soul forces of a person who eats a lot of meat are not engaged sufficiently in the digestion process – they only have to go through one stage: transforming the animal into the human. However, if we eat plant food, we have to carry out the transformation from the vegetable to the animal, and then from the animal to the human; we go through a double sequence of stages, and in so doing we employ forces which otherwise remain dormant. But these forces, if unused, don't just remain idle; they draw into the organism processes that manifest as depository conditions, like calcinosis.

Reading about these complex processes in popular writings, people tend to attribute this to an excess of uric acid. Yet there is a simple principle at work here: if I eat plants, I have to go through a two-stage process; if I eat animal products, I only have a one-stage process. It would, however, be misguided to eat only plants just because this utilises more forces. *There should be no sectarianism in nutrition, no single valid point of view.* We need to cultivate insight so that we gradually learn to discern whether we have sufficient forces available to be able to take in plant nourishment and to digest it consistently, or whether we are so tired and weakened that we don't have the necessary forces at our disposal to digest vegetable food.

It would be misguided for people who don't engage in much conscious mental activity but do a lot of physical work, to live only on vegetable food.[5] Doing this would give rise to a peculiar condition. Such individuals would develop strange symptoms of apathy and become tired, since through a preoccupation with the digestive process, through the extra effort needed to process the plant food, they would have no surplus forces to stay awake. Rudolf Steiner pointed out that people who don't engage in much conscious mental activity should avoid a vegetarian lifestyle.[6] People living exclusively on vegetable food while not engaging in mental activity would eventually develop degeneration of the brain.[7] Everybody can experience a feeling of lightness and elation after eating a vegetarian meal in contrast to a meat meal. If one is sufficiently active on a conscious level, one will not experience heaviness and sleepiness or the need to lie down after consuming a vegetarian meal.

If someone stops eating meat and starts eating vegetable foods, physiological disturbances, such as tiredness and exhaustion, will be experienced for the first few weeks. However, once the corresponding forces in their organism have been harnessed and become effective, the situation will have moved forward considerably. Yet it would be completely misguided to think that to be a decent human being it is essential to live on vegetable food. Eating killed animals is after all supported by the Bible. The human being is placed *in the midst* of nature and has to be able to take responsibility for taking in the widest variety of substances. Nevertheless, personally I am convinced that a meat diet is becoming increasingly unsuited for our time. Apart from those engaged in the heaviest manual labour, most people nowadays should be able to manage well on suitably prepared vegetable food. Beyond this, a meat diet should be considered necessary only when medically prescribed.

Sadly, however what exists nowadays as vegetarianism does not usually bear witness to a proper understanding of what is entailed in the suitable preparation of vegetarian meals. Although meat may have been eliminated, vegetarian meals are often prepared as if they were meat. A vegetarian meal has to be prepared completely differently from a mixed diet. Indeed, if one has not learnt how to use the various culinary herbs, spices and condiments, including the art of combining them, there is little point in attempting vegetarian cookery – and even less in restricting oneself to a vegetarian diet. We would not be satisfied by the result since everything tastes bland. We might then come to feel that we would rather give up the cause and revert to eating meat. If the cook lacks the knowledge to prepare vegetarian meals, the outcome will not confer the necessary sense of well-being; vegetarian cookery requires a completely different approach from conventional cookery.

If we frequent restaurants in Paris and order anything on the menu, we will experience how the French have retained a traditional knowledge of foods. Although this does not provide anything new, it means that individual dishes are served separately, one after the other. The meat is served first; that is a meal in itself; then follows another dish, and the food that is served is prepared in a special way. The French would never dream of serving root vegetables, such as carrots or salsify, with celeriac, or to use gentian root as a condiment, as they know that this will enhance the root element, while it actually needs to be balanced. They will add aniseed to a root vegetable as it is a seed, and the root and the seed together constitute something like a whole plant. The French have retained a natural feeling for this but we need to renew a similar feeling again on the basis of insight.

Only when our thinking has become re-enlivened will we be able to adopt a vegetarian lifestyle. Nowadays housewives talk to each other, complaining that they never know what to cook, because all imagination with regard to cooking has been lost. It is hard to imagine anything nicer than to cook imaginatively, to cook the most wonderful dishes that would make people healthy, born from an overview of nature. There is really no need for people to stand at a loss at the market, worrying desperately about what to cook. There are literally hundreds of things we can cook by way of vegetables and condiments, etc. We need to discover how beautifully the individual ingredients could be prepared, to provide food suited to people's individual needs. In advocating this, I am not proposing to turn everyone into a gourmet.

Now I would like to consider the human being in a threefold nature. In the metabolic system we live with our will, in the middle system with the rhythmic feeling and in the head organ-isation with our thinking. Now the following question arises from this: if we take an animal, a plant or a mineral substance into our organism, are these then distributed evenly to the head, the middle and the metabolic system, or is it rather the case that mineral, plant and animal substances nourish quite different regions of the human being?

The effects of all foods of animal origin are really con-fined to the building up and breaking down processes in the metabolic-limb system. All meat and animal fats only enter the viscous surging and weaving processes in our lower organism. The limb and metabolic system is stimulated by animal food that is taken in, be it pork, beef, wild fowl or poultry. Any substance of animal origin does not go beyond just this lower metabolic system, the realm of viscous activity, and does not rise up any further in the organism. Only when plants are added to the diet, when we get used to eating vegetables, salads, fruit, roots, when we obtain our nutrition from the whole realm of nature, do we reach the next level. Wherever plants are introduced into the human organism, they are not only digested within the solid and liquid sphere. Plants impact on the middle system. When looking at a plant, we can imagine how it is immersed in the sphere of air and light and yet also takes up the earthly being; in this wonderful interaction which holds sway in the plant in such a mysterious way, the plant builds its own organism out of the realm that is permeated by light, air and water. The plant represents for nature nothing other than what lung and heart represent for our own organisation. The blood streams in from below and the breathing from above, both flowing together within the middle organisation; this airy and watery realm, this interplay with the blood circulation, in heart and breathing, in the lung, in the middle organisation, constitutes the sphere which is able to be receptive to plant foods.

We may become aware of breathing differently depending on whether we consume either vegetables or meat and animal fats. Food of animal origin tends to make us feel heavy; everything is as if pulled down into a dark realm of decomposition.[8] When we add plant foods, higher forces are stimulated, not only those that flow and have life, but also those that work in us as breathing process. This does not only apply to the air; just as the external air is permeated by light, the inner air is permeated by the soul element. This activity is awakened and fired up through everything we take in by way of vegetable food. It lives in all the rhythms of our organism. Anything of an animal nature lives in the dull, watery and earthy metabolism down below, while in the airy, living interplay of the upper and the lower, in this soul-permeated airy space of our body, we take in the plant, bringing the environment, the plant, together with our own being, and in this way stimulating the cosmic nutrition stream.

Mineral substances pass upwards to the head organisation. Now, a very special organ, the pineal gland, is situated in our head. Between birth and death this gland forms certain calcium deposits. Here substances that have been ingested are crystallised out; minerals are carried upwards and are deposited. We will understand how essential such a process is when we realise that these calcium deposits are only found in people whose waking consciousness unfolds in the normal developmental pattern, and that individuals with certain learning disabilities lack such calcium deposits.[9] This implies that those with a more dream-like consciousness also manifest differences in their calcium metabolism, that the intake of mineral substance in our organism has a vitalising effect on consciousness. Minerals are necessary for our head organisation just as plant substances are necessary for our rhythmic organisation. Implicit in our capacity to discern these forces consciously is the call to discriminate between these different levels in our food.

Traditionally a distinction has always been made between red and white meat. Red meat is beef and white meat is veal and poultry. However, this differentiation is not sufficient for a truly rational approach. If you look at a cow or an ox, a chicken, a pigeon or a goose, you have entirely different qualities before you. A cow or an ox is altogether an earth-bound animal, and it has developed in a particularly strong way the stomach and intestines that are characteristics of the ruminant. These are developed in an incredibly plastic and powerful way. The digestive system is dominant in all cattle, their head hanging somewhere there. [König was possibly drawing at this point; however, it is more likely – and typical for him when describing animals – that he expressed the animal forms through movement and gesture.] Birds are just the opposite. They are animals without a large intestine and therefore cannot retain the products of digestion. This results from the fact that they cannot consolidate the end products of digestion; essentially they don't digest at all in the real sense. However, they develop feathers, which enable them to fly and hover.

An animal which lives in the realm of the air is completely different from an animal that lives on the earth, which is why the meat of a bird is something completely different from that of a cow. Everything that contains the animal element in its inner nature acts exclusively on the lower organisation. However, it is important to differentiate between beef and poultry. Poultry meat is more easily digested because its whole metabolism is very refined. The muscle fibres in poultry are much more delicate than those of beef. They are not only thinner but also more delicate, because the whole structure is softer and more refined. It is also not a matter of indifference whether we eat pigeon, duck or goose. Pigeon meat is more easily digested than duck. Everything which flies is lighter, more elevated, more head-like. *A bird is really nothing but a liberated human head.* If you were to take off your head, if you were to remove the super-sensible organisation of your head, it would fly away just like a bird. The reality of this is expressed in many fairy tales. The head is a bird attached to the rest of the human organisation. This is why the genius of Homer or Plato has been depicted in the form of an eagle or a vulture sitting on their shoulder or on their head. What Plato called the *Daimon* is a real bird; it is a head being, just as the cow is a metabolic being. This enables us to understand why bird meat is more digestible than beef and why the meat of a domestic goose, which is land-bound, is harder to digest than pigeon meat.

Let us now turn to the plant. There are many differences in the way individual plant foods need to be cooked and enjoyed. Like animals, plants too do not constitute a homogeneous entity that in this case acts on the middle organisation, as initially described. Here too we find internal differentiation. We can look for example at a seed and follow its progress into the soil, observing how it develops. Two kinds of supersensible forces may initially be discerned within the seed, which then shoot out and manifest sense-perceptibly:

- The first one enters the soil and forms the root
- The second one reaches upwards and forms the first rudiments of the stem.

The latter breaks through the seed in an upward direction and the thrust of the root breaks through in a downward direction. When the plant then begins to branch out and the individual leaves and the stem develop, and when new leaves are formed, the plant becomes ever more unearthly. Particularly at the moment the bud begins to form, the plant leaves the earthly realm; initially the rhythmic unfolding of the leaves is halted; the flower is formed and begins to radiate; these flowers are much less earthly, much less solid, much more dissipating than leaves and roots. For the plant to reach the flower stage implies that it is exuding substances because it is so delicate in its colour and form as to almost dissolve. As we move up the plant, it becomes ever finer and more delicate, almost blown away.

Eating a flower is a completely different matter from eating a root, which by nature is sunk into the ground. Roots are rich in bitter mineral extracts, like for example gentian root. It is so strong that the moment it enters your mouth you can immediately identify it. Soups made from roots have a strong flavour, particularly if you have made it exclusively with salsify, swede (rutabaga) and other root vegetables. Many people have an aversion to such soups, sometimes even to the extent of being unable to swallow them as they taste so bitter. There are some children who resist eating certain roots.

Picture to yourself acrid, bitter, hard roots and then, in contrast, picture flowers, not hard and solid, almost as though they might fly away. The flower moves in the direction of sweetness, dispersion, brightness of colour. Only after the plant, having moved through the stages of leaf and flower, has come to an end, does it again form a fruit from the seed. This in turn encompasses the whole plant, now as a singular form. If you happen to travel through the countryside, try observing the landscape and note how apple trees or pear trees, birch trees or oak trees grow. You will notice that in their overall shape trees repeat the form of the fruit. An apple bears the essential stamp of the whole apple tree. Similarly, a pear is shaped like the whole pear tree and the oak tree resembles the acorn in its overall shape. We really need to learn to observe the world around us and to develop a discerning consciousness for form and structure in the individual phenomena. The fruit will then be seen to repeat the overall shape of the plant.

The next question we need to ask ourselves concerns the nature and direction of the activity of roots, leaves, flowers and fruits. What happens when eating a leaf salad or a soup made with roots? Leaves affect the rhythmic system; they come closest to the middle of the plant itself, and for this reason Goethe said, 'metamorphosis can be observed in the leaf.' *The leaf is the plant within the plant.* We find this effect in salad vegetables. The root represents the earthy, solid, hard mineral element and affects the head. Eating them has a hardening, strengthening effect on the head organisation. Flowers affect the metabolism. We drink lime blossom tea rather than gentian root tea because flowers, such as lime blossom and elderflower, stimulate the whole metabolism. All flowers stimulate the lower organism, fire up the whole metabolism, and in cases of fever they promote perspiration.

To treat stomach ache, take a few drops of gentian root. In case of indigestion the metabolic activity dominates the more sensory, glandular activity, and if the sensory activity of the stomach is depressed, gentian root is a suitable remedy. In cases of overexcitement, however, take valerian to encourage the radiant resonating activity of the nerves in a downward direction. This implies that the calming effect of lime blossom tea is achieved, through stimulating the metabolism. Camomile acts on the stomach; yet if we give too much to children, it may cause cramps. This means that with children it may be advisable only to use camomile as a stomach compress.

It is important not to approach these matters in a purely abstract way by stating: roots always work on the head, etc. There are many possible variations, and these need to be studied. Let us consider one particular group, the cruciferous plants; this encompasses all kinds and gradations from flower to root, always somewhat the same and always somewhat different. For example, cauliflower, Brussels sprouts, kale, Savoy cabbage, green cabbage, kohlrabi and swede (rutabaga) manifest essentially the same gesture, yet each expresses its own unique metamorphosis within the whole plant. With regard to cauliflower we can say that is not really a flower at all, but it is rather the metamorphosis of a leaf that has almost turned into a flower and therefore acts most strongly on the digestion. In this way we can proceed through the whole cabbage plant until we reach the swede, which is a root. An incredible menu could be put together out of all this. The Brussels sprout is a bud; when the flower is just about to turn into a leaf, we get red cabbage; kohlrabi arises from a thickening of the leaf stalks, and then it precedes right down to the swede.

If you consider vegetables, you will be able to sense whether a particular person has a greater preference for cauliflower or swede. Most people much prefer cauliflower as it exerts its effects on the stomach, while swede does so on the head. For this reason swede and kohlrabi will be good for certain things, actual cabbage for others. Kohlrabi grows above the earth and swedes in the ground. Savoy cabbage is loosely formed and has frayed leaves. We see how within a single family of plants, metamorphosis extends from the flower via the stem right down to the kohlrabi and the swede, and how this understanding can be utilised for nutrition.

The number of leaf vegetables is endless – spinach, lettuce, lamb's lettuce (corn salad), endive, sorrel, nettles, dandelion leaves, to mention but a few. You should try preparing a soup from the first dandelion leaves in order to experience what a beautiful and stimulating food this is. Tarragon is also an important leaf plant.

Root vegetables include carrots, beetroot, celeriac, turnips and parsnips. Asparagus is a bud that has not yet turned into a leaf bud; it has a certain root quality that tends towards the kidneys; it stimulates kidney function and is helpful in cases of deposits in the metabolic system. However, where there is a tendency to kidney stones, caution is advised in its use.

Onions and leeks all grow on top of or just below the surface of the soil; they are thickened root-stalks of a particular kind. What is a leek? Why does it have such a strong smell? Because the flowering tendency, when carried downwards, becomes a pungent aroma in the root. Potatoes grow below ground, but they too are not real roots. If we consider root, leaf and flower in this way, we do indeed encounter an essential quality in the sense that the root acts predominantly on the head organisation, the leaves on the middle organisation – the rhythmic sphere – and the flower on the lower organisation. However, it must be appreciated that the root not only acts on the head but also on the bones, and that flowers not only act on the lower organisation but also on the nerves; camomile in particular acts on the abdominal nerves.

Now let us consider fruits. The human being, considered as a whole system, is permeated by nerves in the solid bones, in the living muscles and in the metabolism; the fourth level of organisation is the blood. It is fruits that particularly affect the blood. And just as the whole human being is mirrored in the blood, the whole plant is mirrored in the fruit, in the flesh containing various forms of seeds. Look at the fruit and then look at the heart with its surrounding blood vessels. In this picture the effect of fruits on the human organism is captured. The heart corresponds to the core with the surrounding flesh.

It is important to distinguish the effect of fruits with stones, which is totally different from that of pomaceous and berry fruits such as raspberries, gooseberries and blueberries. There are also the tropical fruits: bananas, oranges, leading over to pomaceous fruits, such as apples and pears, and further on to the stone fruits, such as plums, apricots, gages, cherries, peaches. Fruits with hard stones comprise a whole range. It is these in particular which act on the upper organisation of our blood. Pomaceous fruits such as apples and pears, with their harmonious structure, affect the middle organisation/system, while berries relate to the lower part of the organism. In berries the stones or pips have been completely dissolved and the flesh predominates. Think of gooseberries, red and blackcurrants, blueberries. It is obvious that the stone element has been overcome. Pomaceous fruits are more contracted, while stone fruits are completely contracted into a stone. You may also be aware that the stones in stone fruits contain traces of poison in the form of prussic acid (hydrogen cyanide). Although it is contained within an organic compound, the stones should not just be consumed indiscriminately. The stones also have a particular taste. This means that we can look at fruits in a threefold way.

Here is a suggested menu:
- Stone fruits for desserts
- Leafy vegetables as a main course
- Roots of the lower region as a starter, for instance different forms of radishes

Why are radishes served with beer in Munich? It is to enable the people there to 'hold down their drink', since radishes stimulate their digestion. Radishes affect the lower organs. Radishes can be likened to the inhabitants of Munich. This is not intended to cast aspersions on these people. I only wanted to give an illustration of the way plants can be viewed.. This differentiation into flowers, leaves, fruits and roots needs to be taken into account when composing a menu, not selecting only plants from the upper realm, but really taking account of the whole human being.

The next question that needs to be considered is the significance of the cooking process against raw food. Why do we cook particular foods? Why do we prefer to eat fruits raw when they are ripe, and roots mostly not raw, and why do we like to steam leafy vegetables? We can understand this if we imagine that the root contains the most minerals, the leaf is in the middle and that the fruits are warmed through by the sun, making cooking superfluous. The root, which was buried in the dark earth, needs to be cooked for a long time. Leaves cannot be cooked for a long time, as they readily disintegrate: we merely need to steam them. And we can easily eat fruits raw. Obviously there are no objections to be raised against raw food. If we eat beetroot and leaves raw, they have a particular effect in the organism. Raw food has therapeutic benefit when we want to stimulate all the forces in the body. An organism encompasses a multitude of activities.

In order to digest a root – particularly if it is an uncooked root plant – many pathways have to be gone through, unlike a banana, which has already been 'cooked' through by the sun. A root lives in the dark earth and needs to be cooked. A diet of raw root vegetables eaten over many days with a therapeutic purpose can lead to a loss of quite a few pounds in weight. This process is not suitable for everybody, however. Raw food has a particular stimulating effect on the metabolism, and these forces are strongly challenged when we eat raw root vegetables.

Generally speaking, a diet confined to raw food cannot be considered universally beneficial: certain people may need to eat meat, others cooked vegetables, or a mixed diet, and yet others raw food. Everyone needs to work out the best diet for themselves and the members of their family. An obese person needs a different diet from a slim one, an alert one from a dreamy one. Such questions will be considered in the next lecture, when we will address appropriate diets for people who are ill or convalescing, and for babies. It is important not only to speak in general terms about the relationship of different foods to human beings, but also about the individuals themselves in their unique makeup – whether they are of a melancholic, phlegmatic, choleric or sanguine temperament, whether the children are constitutionally more large-headed or small-headed; we will also consider the question of whether it is possible to influence child development therapeutically through food.

3 Childhood and Infant Nutrition

Lecture 3, April 1936

By way of introduction to this subject, we will first develop certain general perspectives concerning the nutrition of children and babies.

We have already considered the significance of a meat diet compared to a vegetarian diet. We have also tried to build a comprehensive picture of the essential nature of the various foods we consume: we have characterised the nature of root, fruit, leaf and flower; the different kinds of meat, and we have been able to establish a broad and overarching framework for assessing the fundamental nature of a particular type of food. We have made it clear that diet is not simply a matter of calculating the calorific value of carbohydrates, proteins and fats. A qualitative evaluation of foods should also be cultivated, addressing the inner character of the different plants we eat, the way they are shaped, as well as how our own individual constitutional predisposition stands in relationship to the foods nature provides for our nourishment.

Our topic today really constitutes a sad chapter of present day human history, because I have the impression that there is hardly any realm in which so many sins are committed as in the nutrition of children and babies.

It is understandable that a mother is proud if her child is plump, and that she is sad if it is thin. When speaking to mothers everywhere – not only in Germany – we encounter the mistaken notion that a child needs to eat a lot, that it needs to put on weight. Children are only considered viable when they have plump cheeks and have put on sufficient weight.

This is a completely misguided attitude. We should not judge the health of children by their weight. The variety of foods given to children has escalated enormously. It is unbelievable that a physician should advise giving a child of nine or ten months of age meat and broth made from bones. The child gains weight, and so the doctor's prescription is judged to have been successful. Children of three, four and five months are given red wine to give them rosy cheeks. I am sure such practices are still encountered today. When these children grow up, when they reach 25, 26, 27 years of age, they often become restless and fidgety, to such an extent that they are unable to focus their attention. You can visit a beer garden and watch young children drinking beer and wine together with their parents.[1] People really have no idea of the way errors made regarding the nutrition of children affect their whole future life. Babies in the delicate early months of life are given unsuitable food because people have no idea and no insight into what is appropriate for such an infinitely delicate being. In Silesia, my former home, it is quite common for twelve-, thirteen-, fourteen-months-old children to sit at table with their parents and to join in a meal of sausages as well as much else. We need to be clear about the fact that there is not much difference between a mother on a low income giving her child sausages and a doctor prescribing meat.

I will attempt to give an introduction to the fundamentals of what is involved in this realm so that you can form some idea of how to inform and advise on nutrition for babies from the perspectives of anthroposophy.

Fortunately, since the [First World] War mothers' milk has come to be recognised as the essential nutrition during the early months of life. But even here one sometimes comes across unbelievable excesses. Recently I saw a nine-year-old child weighing

60 kilos (130 lb) and the mother had not stopped breastfeeding him until the age of fifteen months. It is tempting to breastfeed for this length of time because it is pleasant for the mother, but that does not mean that it is necessarily good for the child. A child certainly needs to be breastfed until there is the first hint of the milk teeth breaking through. This can be around the fifth or sixth month. Up to that time a child needs to be predominantly breastfed. Indications stating that this should be done five to six times a day are correct. Nights should be quiet if possible, even if the baby does not manage it during the first few weeks. Eventually most children will get used to sleeping through from 10 o'clock in the evening to 6 o'clock in the morning. Depending on both mother and child, feeds need to be increased gradually, although there can be no fixed norms, until about the fifth or sixth month. Obviously there are children who need to be given supplementary feeds from the fourth month.[2] If for example a child is suffering from constipation during its third, fourth, sixth month, this is an indication that supplementary feeds are required.

If a child is constipated during the first year of life this is a sign that this being is reluctant to embrace its body, especially with respect to its lower organism. A baby is an infinitely delicate being, whose soul and spiritual existence does not yet reach the earth. It does not engage on that level and as a result develops constipation. If one then administers a little fruit juice, tangerine juice, orange juice – with a teaspoon – mixed with a small amount of malt and sugar, this will pass.[3] A child between one-and-a-half and two years of age should not be given beet sugar. There are three kinds of sugar: On the basis of what has been said previously, we can understand that beet sugar is derived from a root, cane sugar from the realm of stem and leaf, while fruit sugar is really derived from the supra-earthly realm. Therefore, if such a baby does need to be given sugar, the very best choice is fine, gentle cane sugar, because this is the most harmonious and natural form. If you give the child a half to a whole teaspoon of fruit juice mixed with cane sugar, you will notice how gradually the constipation, signifying a reluctance to touch the earth, will generally subside completely.

Now the question arises as to which foods should first be given to supplement breast milk. To understand this question we really need to enter into the nature of milk. Mother's milk is really one of the most wonderful products in existence. You only need to consider how it is that immediately after birth mother's milk begins to flow, having a harmonious composition unlike anything else in nature. It has a distribution of protein-metal-mineral-fat substances in a ratio unlike that from other sources. Whether cow's milk is used or any other kind of milk, there is not a single natural or man-made product that can replace mother's milk. A man such as Paracelsus, who still possessed traditional insights, spoke of mother's milk as a supersensible being ('the good mummy'), transmitted by the mother to the milk. We are justified in thinking that through mother's milk a great deal flows into the child; indeed, it is the first enticement offered by the earth to the supersensible being. This mother's milk is holding a conversation with the soul-spiritual being of the child, saying: 'Do come down into the body and connect yourself with the earth!' This is the supersensible being that is continually speaking to the child. Obviously, beautiful as well as less beautiful things pass from mother to child, but the important thing is that milk should be administered directly. It is the first incentive to that part of the child's being that is still entirely living and breathing with the soul-spiritual realm, which also surrounds the bodily organisation.

Babies' development begins with lifting their head, then lifting themselves up gradually, focusing the eyes, grasping hold of objects, possibly one of the most marvellous processes we are able to behold as human beings. Do not miss the opportunity to observe a baby in all these processes. If we observe this in the right way, we not only experience the most significant aspects of human and earth existence, but through observing the way children begin to grasp hold of objects, lift up their head, raise themselves up, sit up, we may be able to assess the way developing children are likely to make a connection to life. Such observations build the foundations from which therapeutic approaches in helping and guiding the incarnating child are derived. It is of significance whether children sit up with a jolt or whether they lift up their head gently and gradually sit up; whether they proceed from sitting to crawling or immediately to walking. This makes a tremendous difference. When children learn to walk, some will immediately put down their heels, while others walk on their toes. This is not arbitrary, but immensely significant for the whole human being. Young children walking on their toes will take hold of the world in a more delicate way than those who put their heels down. We need to observe this in order to develop reverence for the eternal individuality that is trying to enter the earthly world through the child. These seemingly incidental remarks help to build an essential context for considering questions of child nutrition.

During the sixth month one should begin to give children supplementary food – depending on the rate of their development, whether they have started sitting up, whether the first tooth has appeared in the lower or upper jaw – mothers need to observe this carefully and to act out of maternal intuition. Milk is really the product of the most subtle processes. Dr Steiner pointed out that the closest thing to milk is fruit that has been warmed through by the sun.[4] This picture is really crucial. If in this realm – pictorially speaking – we endeavour to put children on the earth immediately by giving them carrot juice, this may miss the mark or even do harm. If the first supplementary food we give children after milk is carrots, the effect of this will be to draw the soul-spiritual being down to the earth.[5]

We only need to look at plants – at leaves, flowers, fruits – to realise that fruits are closest to milk. For most children the right thing will be to move from milk first to fruits and from there to flowers and gradually to leafy vegetables. Only when children are able to tolerate these should we proceed to root vegetables. In addition one can give them something from the realm of seeds, for instance, some flour. One can begin to feed them porridge made from flour, semolina or a little rice. This is the ideal sequence in which to proceed, and it will generally prove in some way beneficial. One could use one's imagination; semolina need not only be prepared with milk, but one might add some orange juice, or one might add some spinach to sago.[6] Actually it is not advisable to feed spinach at an early age. One should be very restrained in the use of spinach because it contains iron, and avoid giving it on its own but rather mix it with other foods – then children will get used to it. It is the most delicate matter to gain a proper understanding of a baby in its digestion and to carry out everything in the best way. It is not the body you are guiding, but within the digestion you are trying to guide the spiritual being out of the realm of fairy tale, out of the supersensible realm down to the earth.

The moment children begin to stand and take their first steps – and this may surprise you – you may proceed to allowing them fats. However, refrain from offering them butter before they have gained the ability to stand up, because fat is so much more difficult to digest. It would be out of the question to give children meat broth or eggs. I would like to point this out at the outset, so that you can bear in mind the effect of eggs. Eggs are really only suitable for older children, that is, more for adults. Young children should really only be given eggs on medical advice. Consider what an egg actually is. When people refer to a vegetarian diet, they usually associate this with the consumption of quantities of eggs. Yet eggs have nothing to do with vegetarianism.

An egg has a hard outer shell, and inside is the white of the egg and the yolk. What does this indicate? Although we don't feed the shell to children, whenever we use eggs we should then dry the shells in the oven, as they constitute the best calcium preparation. If children have intestinal worms at the age of five or six, we can grind eggshells, mix them with carrots and feed them to the children; this will get rid of their worms. The shell is the substance that draws all the earthly forces out of the egg. This is set aside, just as in the case of the human being the skull contains the receptive brain. What remains inside the hard eggshell is the egg white and the yolk, and these are devoid of any hardening forces, of any root forces. And when you give a child eggs to eat you are doing the opposite to what the child is doing. The child is trying to gradually descend, first into the head, then into the middle system, and finally to take hold of the lower organism. If we give a child eggs, the spiritual aspect is rejected slightly, it remains excarnated. The effect on the body is then like allowing a ball to drop to the ground. The nutritional value is not the primary consideration. The essential aspect is that eggs loosen the supersensible organisation and repel it. There are occasions when it may be advisable to give an egg to thin, intellectual children, who are drawn to engaging with machines, as eggs slow the tendency to descend to earth prematurely, but otherwise refrain from giving children too many eggs.

If children have gained a balanced upright position in relation to the forces of earth, one may let them eat a little butter, a little oil, and accustom them to the most diverse combinations of foods, such as roots, leaves and fruits. There is a rich choice of boiled and steamed foods, but you should protect your children from deep-fried foods until the seventh year. Deep-fried foods are amongst the hardest to digest, as they make demands of the digestive system that young children are not yet able to fulfil. The head is the centre of the young child's being – its whole organisation is still contained in the head, and the digestive forces can only be engaged gradually and gently, thus enabling them to establish themselves harmoniously in the earthly realm. There can also be no question of children needing to eat meat before the age of fourteen, unless they are ill; in fact I actually consider it inappropriate to do this.

Let us for the moment stay with young children. Up to the

third year a mixed (vegetarian) diet is appropriate. When they have reached the third year and developed the faculty of memory, that is, when they are able to recall their own outer and inner experiences, only then is it appropriate to allow them to sit at table and eat adult food. However, alcohol, beer, meat, deep-fried foods and mushrooms are to be avoided. Mushrooms are plants lacking any sun forces. They have sunk to the earth. You only have to observe them to notice how on the one hand they tend towards the poisonous and on the other towards a kind of sexual function. Don't give children mushrooms before their fourteenth year – they don't have a positive effect before that age.

From this kind of approach you may get some idea of the essential key to nutrition for babies and children. We are trying as much as possible to facilitate the engagement of soul life with the sphere of matter. This is a tragic process: the soul being arrives in the realm of earth, of gravity; it experiences its first encounter with death, with the hardness of substances. This should not come as a shock but should take place as gently and lovingly as possible. For this reason a child's first supplementary food should be fruit, moving on to flower, leaf and root vegetables, in that order. This has proved amazingly successful. I have administered rose leaf juice with the addition of a small amount of elderflower juice to a seven to eight-month-old child. In this way we are able gently to draw down the soul being of the child – we can do justice to the soul of the child that is descending to earth.

If we now follow children up to their seventh year and study them – of course we can observe distinct features in all children – we find in broad outline two kinds of children. We are now going to address this differentiation only in broad outline in the form of a schematic picture in order to give maximum scope to maternal imagination.

One group of children is characterised by a small head; they tend to have dark hair, are very awake and interested in the world, are able to count by the age of three or four without having been taught, begin to be interested in the names of the individual letters, etc., and are very keen to take their toys apart as they like to discover how they work. These children are frequently very fidgety, easily jumping from one impression to another. These are the children who continually ask 'why?' and who as early as age two-and-a-half or three begin to ask why spinach is green, etc.

Children of the other kind are characterised by a large head; they are mostly fair-haired, quiet, ask few questions, are not easily excitable and are endowed with strong imagination. They can talk to themselves for hours, playing with a sock. They are able to experience a whole fairy tale world in this sock. Therefore it is much better to give these children very simple toys, not the complicated ones customary today. It is nonsense to give children a painted doll with naturalistic hair and eyes to help them sleep better. Nothing is then left to their imagination. Offer children a suitable piece of wood with a piece of old rag, and then the imagination can begin to play with the wood.

The fair children who are more inclined to be reticent develop a strong imagination. Why is their head so large? Because the imagination has not yet found its way from the embryonic state to the earth. During the fifth and sixth month the embryo is essentially a head supporting some minimal appendages, and only in the course of development does the relative size of the head decrease – it is not that the head gets smaller but that the rest of the organism increases in size. This makes the head appear relatively smaller. Large heads retain more of a relationship to the pre-earthly condition, while small heads gravitate more to the earthly. Children with large heads tend more towards the volatile and are likely to be fair-haired, while the small-headed children tend more towards solidification. In fair-haired children the sulphuric processes predominate in their organism. This makes for fantasy and in extreme cases even for lying. In small-headed children the iron process is predominant, which has a densifying effect, tending towards melancholy, and manifesting an affinity to the earthly.[7]

What should our nutritional approach be with respect to both constitutional types? Large-headed children benefit from a diet of root vegetables, such as carrots, beetroot and salsify, which support the mineralising tendencies. It is the mineral constituents that help in consolidating the formation of the head organisation – they complete the head formation process, densifying it and therefore inclining it more towards the earth, whereas foods derived from the flower enliven the metabolism. Small, fidgety children, particularly those who suffer from metabolic weaknesses such as diarrhoea and bed-wetting, have difficulty controlling their lower organism. In these children we need to stimulate the metabolic life forces. The essential therapeutic gesture with large-headed children is their need to be consolidated, so that they become more formed, more shaped. We may contrast small-headed children with their slightly narrow horse-like heads with the large-headed ones with their broad heads and their flat foreheads. Small-headed children not only need protecting from the effects of root vegetables as foods but also from the effects of root-like thoughts. One should avoid having conversations about life issues with them as one would with an adult, but one should rather lead them into a fairy-tale world and give them appropriate nourishment for the soul as well as for the body. For them this will consist of fairy tales and a fruit diet. With large-headed children, however, you may well speak more freely about earthly matters and give them root vegetables to eat.

It is the main task of parenting to promote health in this way and to develop a sense for the best nutritional approach so that the child's constitutional predisposition does not become more pronounced leading to an illness; so that the small-headed child does not develop diarrhoea, and the large-headed one adenoidal congestion causing recurring tonsillitis and sore throats. Small-headed children are also more inclined to develop appendicitis. An appropriative type of nutrition can be preventative on both accounts.

Children up to around the age of seven should not be given

the usual type of adult drinks. Black tea is harmful. At most a coffee substitute made from barley malt is acceptable; hot chocolate should only be given on medical advice. Cocoa inclines children to density and heaviness so that they become terribly earthbound. In order to understand what I mean – and it is best to point this out at the outset – you need to picture for yourself a hot chocolate party, a coffee party and a tea party. Then you will realise what we are dealing with here.

Cocoa and chocolate are frequently drunk on birthdays. As you sink into your chair, you experience how you sink more deeply into your metabolism with every sip, and finally you find yourself sitting among a lot of cocoa bellies. People become so heavy that they are no longer able to sit up properly; they become so occupied with their metabolism that they are no longer inclined to any conversation.

Tea is a completely different matter. In former times, when there were still true diplomats, it was their most favoured drink. When they were sitting together discussing their diplomatic affairs – this needed to be done in a skilful and lively manner – they would drink tea. Tea promotes imagination, lifts us a little bit above earthly affairs. This is permissible for adults but not appropriate for children.

Now we come to coffee. Imagine a coffee party, a coffee house. There we find the type of persons who need to make an effort to express themselves logically, and be logical in matters relating to other people, linking one fact to another. Coffee promotes wakefulness. We can of course also link other ideas together logically. The overall effect of coffee is that it separates out the physical organisation, freeing up thoughts and associations. This is the reason that many people enjoy drinking coffee, and we can understand why this is so if we take account of these dynamics.

I would emphatically advise against exposing children to these, but this advice will only be followed if people can recognise for themselves what the effects really are. Up to the age of seven you should also protect children from excessive intake of fats, meat, eggs, from frequent consumption of tomatoes and (less drastically) cucumbers, as also from alcohol, tea, coffee and cocoa.

When the children then enter school around their seventh year, in the course of undergoing their second dentition, a new developmental phase begins. The first seven-year phase constitutes the phase of imitation. It is nonsensical to attempt formal education before the age of seven. Everything that father and mother do is imitated by the child, including thoughts, feelings and speech; children will imitate everything, and if as adults we don't behave appropriately in the presence of children, we will not be capable of imparting appropriate education.

Only with the appearance of the second dentition will children begin to develop independent ideas and thoughts; they may then be formally introduced to arithmetic, reading and writing. Concurrently children begin to develop a new relationship to their environment. Dr Steiner described this change in some detail, and his descriptions form the basis of Waldorf education.[8] Children are indeed very different before and after the age of school readiness. Although they will still imitate, they begin to assimilate content independently, now on the basis of adult authority. Between the seventh and fourteenth year, the child needs to be given the opportunity to recognise the inner authority of the teacher and the parents. If children do not experience this, they are likely to retain a scar in later life unless they are able to transform it. This will manifest in the moral sphere, in respectful and considerate behaviour. Between their seventh and fourteenth years children need to be given the possibility to look up to teachers, to parents; this is absolutely essential in view of the different forces out of which the growing child is now living.

Up to the seventh year the children are bound to the formative processes that originate in their head organisation. After the seventh years children begin increasingly to permeate the middle region of their organism, the processes of breathing and pulse, with their soul-spirit being. You can observe the change if you tell a fairy tale to young children and then to school children. Young children will listen with open eyes. After the seventh year the soul life of the child begins to participate directly in the experience. When approaching a gripping passage, the children can turn quite pale, and a lot depends on the way the teacher tells the story. It must not be boring. Then you will notice how the rhythmic organisation with its breathing and heartbeat resonates with the story. In the period between the seventh and the fourteenth year, educators have to do with a being who lives predominantly in the middle region, in the rhythmic system, and the appropriate form of nutrition for children during this age is therefore a mixture of different parts of the plant. Seeds, for instance in the form of baked semolina or flour, all fruits, roots, leaves and most of the flowers can be used as food. Healthy children don't require anything other than food that is derived from plants. Obviously it needs to be varied to make it appetising, but essentially nothing else is needed. Given sufficient imagination, it is possible to manage completely without meat and eggs. Their nutrition may be supplemented with modest amounts of dairy produce, but plant oils are preferable for use in cooking.

It is important to acquire a sense of how children between the seventh and fourteenth year live predominantly in their rhythmic system, and based on what was said in the previous lecture, you will be able to understand why children really benefit from a mainly vegetarian or plant-based diet.

In children of school age their temperament becomes evident: whether melancholic, choleric, sanguine or phlegmatic. What in young children simply manifests more or less as large- or small-headedness now comes clearly to expression in schoolchildren via their temperament. The temperaments are connected in an essential way with our whole physical nature. Their respective characteristics correspond with the way the organism has been endowed with life forces. This is something we are born with, and we all know how difficult it is to transform our temperament, even in the course of a whole lifetime, to abandon our phlegmatic tendency or to restrain our choleric temperament. It is not easy to do this because it is thoroughly inherent in us. Something we were born with, and have helped to shape out of our previous earthly incarnation, manifests more or less between the seventh and fourteenth year. It may be helpful to balance out these temperaments a little through nutrition. We can influence every child in this way, but don't approach this too rigidly. All four temperaments are always present in every individual, but generally one of them will predominate. We can give children a mixed diet, but we should try once a day to prepare a meal specifically tailored to their particular temperament.

What do we mean by phlegmatic, choleric, melancholic and sanguine? How would you describe a melancholic child? Which forces need to be strengthened in this organism, and which in the other ones? Melancholic children are usually thin, skinny, insufficiently relaxed, they may tend to be fixed, bony and not feel at home in the world; they manifest an underlying unhappiness. The earthly forces are working excessively strongly. One can clearly experience that the bodily nature predominates over the other parts of the human being, over the life forces, the soul, the 'I'. Such children cannot readily fit in socially because the earthly element is predominant, resulting from the fact that their supersensible being struggles to establish a relationship to the world through their bodily organisation. Melancholic children need to turn away from the world because their eyes and ears are over-sensitive, brittle, and they find themselves repelled by their bodily organisation and cannot easily develop a relationship to the earth and to the outer world.

Phlegmatic children generally appear pale and plump. The tissues of such lymphatic children tend to lack tone, it is difficult to get them to pay attention – they simply cannot get a grip on it. Here the metabolic system, the watery element, predominates. Everything is in flux, possibly also congested, but in such a way that the fluid is not being sufficiently propelled forward by the wind of the soul element; the wind and the air are not at play within the child's soul. The water flows sluggishly as if about to come to a standstill, and these children are not at all able to penetrate their fluid processes with the force of their supersensible being. It may sometimes be helpful – and preferably through nutrition – to encourage them to become angry and thereby bring their water organisation into movement. Such children benefit from bitter herbs, sour-tasting foods, spices (though not pepper or paprika), anise seed, caraway seed, parsley, marjoram, chervil, lemon. They will often suffer from recurrent colds. They benefit from raw food because this has a stimulating effect. Milk, dumplings, foods made with flour, and potatoes are best avoided. Dry raw foods, very stimulating colourful foods such as beetroot, radishes, hot spices and lettuce dressed with some lemon are the most suitable for phlegmatic children. They may well initially reject these foods, but they will take to them in the long run. Instinctively they would much prefer eating dumplings and sausages because these don't require much effort, but if they are encouraged, and their appetite for these other types of food is stimulated, it is possible to intervene in a healing and transforming manner through nutrition.

Melancholic children benefit from sweeter foods, including flowers. They need to be loosened up in their lower organisation, to go through processes that engage the fiery element. They should be encouraged to eat tropical fruits, which convey to them the forces of the sun. If you give melancholic children lots of tropical fruits, you will notice that they begin to become warmer and more open. This only applies to children; it is a completely different matter in adults. The soul of the adult has become emancipated from the body; children have not achieved this yet, and so we have to support them in this task.

In choleric children the head often appears compressed between the shoulders, the middle organisation is compressed and seems ready to burst open. In such children it is the warmth organism that does not function in a balanced way. It overpowers the other parts. The 'I' dominates in the soul element, in the life forces and the physical body, often explosively. How might such children be nourished? They are inharmonious and benefit from food that will stimulate their rhythmic organism: leafy vegetables, spinach, asparagus, cucumbers, pumpkin. Insipid food will not be suitable for them, but pomaceous fruits such as apples and pears, as well as juices and milk, will be. Salt will not be beneficial.

In sanguine children, especially in the fidgety ones who flit from one thing to the other, who are compelled to learn, to play, to run, and who seem to have the whole world inside them, the airy organism is excessively developed. The soul element or astral body will then tend to lack the guidance of the I-organisation, which is why the child sways to and fro, rushing from one impression to the other. What might we offer such children as food? We need to address and guide their power of concentration and nurture their warmth organism. We need to give them flour-based foods, dumplings, pasta, peanuts, firm wholemeal or rye bread, stimulating the chewing activity. Heavy foods, hearty flour-based foods are indicated, preferably sweet rather than spiced, salty or sour. Such children may even eat mushrooms without problems, as they incorporate too much light anyhow, and can benefit from sinking down into earthly stillness. They may also eat heavy foods without suffering ill effects. In principle one could give a healthy sanguine child standard Prague plain fare (excluding the meat and cabbage, of course): this fare will have a positive effect

To sum up we can say:

- the earth element is predominant in the melancholic,
- the watery element in the phlegmatic,
- the fiery element in the choleric,
- the air element in the sanguine.

Let us now look at the temperaments.[9] In educating school children, we need to be on the alert and pay attention to nutrition. There will be children who during their school years suddenly become thin and shoot up, growing very fast, while others stay plump and round. If we investigate this, we notice that such developments are not solely dependent on the constitution of the children but also on that of the teacher. This does not imply that if the teacher is thin, so will the children be, but one can observe that if the teacher makes high demands on the memory, the children becomes thin, with sudden spurts of growth. Parents may be able to observe this, and need to intervene through nutrition. Occasionally, teachers make too few demands on the memory of small and plump children, appealing too strongly to their imagination. Both extremes can to some extent be balanced out therapeutically by relieving the pressure on the memory of the skinny child and challenging the memory capacity of the plump child. This can be a real therapy; setting obese and plump children memory tasks will stimulate their growth forces. If possible, material particularly suitable for memorising by children should be used. Tall, thin children will need to be relieved of memory work and encouraged to engage in artistic activity, such as painting with watercolours on wet paper. Stimulating their imagination will help them to develop rosy cheeks.

All these measures can be supported through nutrition, and I have already indicated how this can be done. The tall, thin child needs to eat fruit – hot fruit soups as a main meal have a place, as we need to stimulate their warmth processes from within. It is important to develop a sense for whether a child should be given more hot or cold foods. Tall and lanky children need predominantly hot foods that will warm them from within. The short, imaginative child should have more cold dishes, not exactly ice cream perhaps, but salad with a lemon dressing, and root vegetables, in such a way that the food has a cooling, contracting effect. We need to guide these children as well as enabling them to adjust to the conditions of life. It is preferable for adults to adjust to the needs of the children rather than the other way round. Both adults and children will fare better as a result. If we pay attention to the child's appropriate nutrition, we will learn to hold back our own needs, and this will promote a certain moral development. It is helpful if a boy feels that his father is eating with him, rather than he with his father.

In the next lecture we will develop an overview of diets appropriate for certain illnesses.

4 Special Diets

Lecture 4, April 1936

It has been the aim of this whole course to provide a certain schematic overview of the subject of nutrition, and we now come to diets for particular illnesses. It is only possible to outline fundamental principles, and it will depend on the intelligence and the heart forces of the listeners or readers whether these guidelines will be followed schematically or endowed with life. Please don't imagine that you will be provided with prescriptive recipes in today's final lecture; that is the province of medicine, and responsibility rests with the doctor or dietician. In speaking about patient nutrition, it is not my intention to go into specific diseases, as this would far exceed our present framework of possibilities. It is, however, the task of the layman to provide appropriate food during illness and convalescence. I would like to speak pictorially in order to provide a framework for your orientation regarding the one or other life situation.

Let us remind ourselves of what was outlined in the first lecture. Every intake of food represents a certain poisoning of the human organism, and all our digestive and metabolic processes represent the opposite, providing the antidote to this poisoning. It is of the essence of every act of nutrition, that time and again we are called upon to exert our own human forces, not only physically but also our soul and spiritual forces in order to counteract the power, substance and gestalt of the foods. It is not the case that some passive intestinal and gastric juices destroy its

105

constituents: we ourselves as creative human beings of a soul-spiritual nature are active in our organism, intervening in every single metabolic and digestive process, having to resist and overcome the outside world that enters us through the food, and to test and hone our own forces.

In order to develop an understanding for patient diets, let us now consider the relationship between a food and a medicine.

During an illness human beings find themselves in a certain condition in which they require specific medical treatment. I am not referring to the usual kind of medicine, for example one that will lower a fever or suppress symptoms, but true medicaments as developed within the anthroposophical school of medical practice. In this context, how is the difference between a food and a medicine to be conceived? I believe I have already addressed this theme two or three years ago but I would like to briefly repeat what I said then for the sake of absolute clarity.[1]

What is the difference – to take a concrete example – between drinking a decoction of gentian root or consuming a regular item of food, such as a potato? Is there really a difference, or is there none? Are medicines foods, and foods medicines? I am asking you seriously to consider in which way one might differentiate the presence of medicines from the presence of foodstuffs in the organism; in which way one might engage with what is, after all, a fundamental distinction. What is the difference between, say, drinking lime blossom tea and eating a piece of meat? What does a medicine bring about in the organism? After all, when we take in food we upset the existing state of equilibrium in the body; this applies equally to medicines and foods. During an illness this balance will already have been disturbed in one way or the other.

A medicine, however, must not be transformed! As soon as a medicine is destroyed, it is no longer effective. The medicine needs to retain its foreignness within the body. It is precisely through this that it is able to make its own forces available to the organism. This is the essential factor in the preparation and manufacture of a medicine. Pharmaceutical chemists have to design processes that ensure the retention and biological availability of the original constituents. A medicine can only be considered as such if it retains its properties for a while in the organism, if gentian root, for example, is not immediately destroyed but retains its activity for a certain amount of time. Its forces remain available to work, say, on the disturbed sensory function of the stomach, and only when the gentian root has been able to unfold its action there, having brought the sensory function into a kind of equilibrium, only then has it fulfilled its task and is destroyed. The remedy needs to remain intact in the body for a certain amount of time. Foodstuffs, however, become poisonous, as can be the case with milk, when they enter the organism on the other side of the digestive tract; then they act either as a medicine or a poison; they retain their own existence, and reactions such as fever are the result.

The fundamental difference between a medicine and a foodstuff is that the latter has to be destroyed, while a medicine must not be, at least not for a certain time.

Now there are certain substances that represent a transition between foods and medicines. What kind of substances are these? They have to be substances that are not quite foods, but neither are they medicines, for example spices and culinary herbs. Why do spices retain their own taste for a much longer period? Because they retain their own constitution for longer, thereby triggering the beginning of a healing process in the organism. There are spices that act very strongly on the stomach and intestine, while others act on our head. They don't always have to be ingested; they can sometimes also be inhaled or smoked. These are not medicines, nor are they foods; this applies, for example, to chervil, marjoram, etc.

There is a gradual transition between the culinary use of herbs and their pharmaceutical use. In the twelfth and thirteenth centuries people cultivated culinary herbs in their gardens. First there were herb gardens, and later medicinal gardens were added. First parsley was grown and then other herbs. The herb garden was always separate from the vegetable garden because in those days people were aware that substances needing to retain their existence in the organism belong to a different order from those that merely exist to be eaten and then destroyed. Basically, foodstuffs are products of nature that exist in order to be destroyed when eaten, thereby undergoing a process of transformation. They are derived from the natural realm and are cultivated and grown in order to be broken down physically after being eaten, thereby allowing the spirit to light up. They are demolished physically so that they may transcend their natural condition, and be raised up to the supersensible, just as, conversely, the supersensible is being materialised.

With respect to nutrition the key factor when nursing those who are ill is that we can only speak about caring, and not about treatment. It is most important to make sure *that the effect of any medicine is not disturbed through inappropriate food.* If we have to provide food for acutely ill patients – we will speak about the chronically sick later – be they children or adults, the most important thing to bear in mind is not to interfere with the action of the medicine, and not to adversely influence the course of the illness.

If there were a single piece of advice I could offer, it would be the following: in acute cases it is better not to give any food at all if you are not sure what would be appropriate. A child or an adult can easily go without food for one or two days, and this guideline would best serve the course of the illness. It is better to withhold food from an acutely ill person, even if it is a young child. This is not a barbaric punitive measure, but a correct one! Believe me, there is no point in overburdening an organism with digestion and metabolism when it is busy sustaining a temperature of 39° to 40°C (94–96°F) for the whole day. It simply does not make sense to do this. I would like to emphasize that I am only speaking about acutely ill people. If you have a sick child, allow it to fast for a day. Fasting means no solid food. However, a person running a temperature must not be allowed to go thirsty.

What are suitable drinks for feverish children? Lemon – if they don't have a sore throat, otherwise they will cry! I would refrain from giving any complex or exotic juices – rather they should be plain, perhaps some fresh orange juice for example; milk is generally too heavy. We forgot to discuss the place of almond milk in baby nutrition – marshmallow tea *(Althaea officinalis)* is recommended for coughs. But the most wonderful and cheapest of all is peppermint! Made from the leaves, it is the most cooling tea and the ideal drink for a fever, because it cools without draining forces from the organism. This applies both to children and adults. You can also mix peppermint tea with lemon balm and lemon. In the case of fever, the tea should be administered slightly on the cool side.

If feverish children are hungry, what should you give them to eat? Seeds affect the lower organism. In the case of diarrhoea, the best thing is a grated raw apple, one raw apple five times a day. You may be surprised that the effect is not the opposite – that is what tends to be assumed. One can offer lemon and all kinds of other fruit compote, which are marvellous because they are cool. Then you can offer a biscuit or rusk to go with it, and that will be plenty. Don't give any more, unless specifically advised by a doctor. But be careful: under no circumstances should meat broth or eggs be given. We need to keep reiterating that eggs only have a place in young children's diets in exceptional circumstances. They are among the foods that are hardest to digest. I would advocate starting a crusade against eggs. In cases of fever, in acutely ill children, eggs should only be used in minimal amounts in dishes made with flour, and even then, the yolks are best avoided.

One can give children toast or rusks. But meat or anything fried in fat or oil should be avoided; only small quantities of food should be given at a time. Furthermore, as varied as diets should be in health, as simple should they be in illness; only one kind of food should be given at any one meal. If two or three kinds of food are prepared, then they need to be given separately. Children are very sensitive to mixtures of food, especially when they are not yet quite recovered. Each dish should be served separately and prepared in a simple manner. In cases of fever, cool foods are preferable. It is important for patients that the nutrition process remains in the background, and that they should only receive what is essential; in this way we enable the medicines to unfold their own activity. It is the case that unnecessary quantities of food undermine the therapeutic action of remedies. You can also imagine how as a doctor one has not only to choose which remedy to give the patient, but also the optimal dosage.

Inappropriate nutrition can undermine the efficacy of any medicine, because it challenges the organism when its forces should actually remain engaged in the healing process. Let us now return to the question of nutrition during an acute illness: When the patient has got over the acute phase of the illness and enters the stage of convalescence, the scene that confronts a doctor may give cause for concern: The whole family is standing around the bed, everyone having brought an item of food which the patient may feel obliged to eat. Now in reality the patient has come through a particular crisis of destiny – for every illness constitutes such a situation; when that has passed, we may give a sigh of relief. But those healing forces, which have been called upon for a very particular task, are at risk of becoming overwhelmed by the weight of an excessive supply of food. Have you ever observed children convalescing after a bout of scarlet fever or measles, after an inflammation of the kidneys or pneumonia? If you are attentive, you may observe how they are able to unfold completely new traits of character that had not previously been evident. After scarlet fever a child may, for example, begin to draw certain figures or may suddenly ask for plasticine or clay, because every illness may stimulate a breakthrough to a new capacity.

If, however, we consider the convalescent patient merely as an object to be built up with food, we will be suppressing the forces that are trying to be liberated. What the person has gained through the illness – through going through the disease process – will not be able to come to manifestation. You need to look upon a convalescent patient as a being at the beginning of a new descent to the earth, establishing a new connection to the bodily organisation. During the time of recuperation, the worst thing one can do is to overwhelm the recovering patient with a variety of foods. In fact the best thing would be to advise all relatives not to bring anything whatsoever by way of food! Depending on the nature of the illness, it is important to first introduce one particular kind of food. After a fever, for example, one can begin with the harmony of the leafy vegetables: spinach, lettuce, mixed with a little fruit and root vegetables; light bread is also suitable, gradually getting the organism used to managing a normal diet and to employing stronger digestive forces. The results of the illness – I am referring to the destiny aspect that is being liberated – manifest as completely new capacities; these will be lost if a normal diet or even the customary convalescent diet is resumed immediately.

So what sort of diet is considered suitable for patients nowadays – veal, marinated chicken, pigeon, mashed potatoes and such like? This is completely misguided; this is food for old people but not for convalescents. It is always assumed that a convalescent is to be treated like an old person. A person in convalescence needs to be treated like a child, a developing child who is being guided towards the earth – initially exclusively through a vegetable diet.

In recent years important scientific discoveries have been made. Ragnar Berg, working in Dresden, has demonstrated that it is only with a vegetable diet that our whole organism responds with an alkaline reaction.[2] Slogans are bandied about: meat makes the body too acidic. What does this signify? The acidification simply means that through acidic reactions in the urine our whole organism becomes heavy and dark. Berg investigated the breathing, blood and bodily fluids in a variety of pathological conditions and found that blood reacting in an acidic way is somehow thicker than blood displaying an alkaline reaction, that the urine is different and that breathing is lighter with a plant diet. Generally a plant diet is beneficial under normal circumstances, but it has even greater virtue during and after an illness. If guided by real insight, one would always avoid giving patients suffering from acute illnesses any kind of meat, both during the illness as well as during convalescence.

111

Meat is the last thing that a sick person is able to tolerate. As long as a sick person or a child needs to be looked after, in my opinion meat should be avoided in the diet.

This is addressing the whole issue of the over-acidification of our organism. However, we will not be able to tackle the problem with the measures customarily employed until the idea of a pure and properly prepared vegetable-based diet begins to be taken seriously – not raw food, but a plant diet that maintains to a certain degree the vitality of our organism. Such a diet will not allow these newly acquired forces to weaken, but will stimulate and renew them. Vitality and a continuous renewal of the organism will be achieved in this way.

For children with bronchitis and a head cold – even when there is no fever – root vegetables and lemon are beneficial. But we should also discuss when honey might be given. Honey is one of the most wonderful products of nature, but we should only use it if we can do so responsibly. Dr Steiner spoke about it in a wonderful way, telling us what the 'land of milk and honey' really is. It is the land where there are healthy children and beautiful old people. If we were to arrange all foods into an entire spectrum, we would place honey on one side of the spectrum and milk on the other. If we study this polarity, then all foods encompassed within this spectrum are from the land of milk and honey.

Dr Steiner said, 'Honey is the milk of the aged.'[3] This is the most beautiful thing that can be said about this substance. It is the appropriate food for old people. (Of course children can also be old and brittle on occasion, in which case they may also benefit from being given honey.) An appropriate characterisation of honey is that it is indicated primarily where there are signs of sclerosis. Honey embodies the most delicate sugar process. The sugar is not only derived from the flower, but is taken up by the bee and processed. It is an enhanced sugar that has passed through an animal species, that the sugar is transformed by bees. Therefore honey counteracts everything by way of sclerosis, darkness, heaviness, desiccation; honey has a place where there is an excess of salt and deposit formation. It has incredible forces that have a lightening effect on the whole organism. It cannot do harm. And milk is the opposite of honey. Milk attracts the soul-spiritual element. Honey draws the hardened organism up to the soul-spiritual sphere in order to enable it to light up and to be permeated with light. That is why the land of milk and honey is the land where there are healthy children and beautiful old people!

Let us return to the subject of bronchitis. Were we to give children only root vegetables and lemon, this would be insufficient. Imagine such children, where everything is streaming. If we were to feed them fruit, they would develop terribly runny noses. Children in this situation should be given dry foods, dry raisins, a little muesli with water, to give them the possibility of restoring their fluid metabolism to its proper place in the organism. A head cold is actually the whole metabolic process rising up to the head organisation, overwhelming the sense organs and the lungs. In bronchitis the diaphragm is, as it were, pulled away between metabolism and respiration, so that the metabolism overwhelms the lungs and floods it with water. This is only a picture, but this is the fundamental nature of the process. So children need to be given foods that help the waters to begin to go down; this is dry food, because it enables the intestines and the metabolism to draw the excess water from the upper to the lower organisation. I am using such typical examples so that you can see how these matters need to be approached.

Dry food is raw uncooked food, and without drinks. Raw food contains a variety of juices while dry food does not. It can easily be mixed with different things. You can give a child puffed rice oat flakes soaked in water and mixed with some dried fruits.

By way of digression, what is a starvation diet or a diet involving abstaining from fluids? You know that for years starvation diets have been tried, and that people have been made to go for two, three and four weeks without food. Diets involving abstention from fluids are employed in certain ways. In Germany there is a sanatorium specifically dedicated to such diets. Sometimes amazing results are achieved by such means, for example with Schroth cures.[4] Or it is according to the motto, 'If it doesn't kill you, it makes you stronger!' One should beware of embarking on a starvation diet to lose weight without medical advice. People have no idea – that is why I am saying this – of the far-reaching changes taking place in any organism starved for more than two or three days. What is normally only achieved with the heaviest meat diet – a complete over-acidification of the body – is achieved by three days of starvation. A complete over-acidification of the organism takes place. At that point the organism begins to consume its own substance, to digest what it has accumulated. Apart from this one has to imagine what kind of responsibility one takes on if – I can say this on the basis of what has been said already – we prevent the cosmic nutrition stream from entering the organism. We would be cutting it off as its flow depends on the fact that we are taking in food in a particular way. The demolition of the food allows the cosmic nutrition stream to enter. We should refrain from embarking on such a cure without medical guidance.

Now you will have heard of the Gerson diet[5] that has produced such marvellous results in cases of tuberculosis, in particular in lupus, skin, bone and joint tuberculosis. In pulmonary tuberculosis the results are debated. The salt that we normally take in directly, is missing in this diet. You know that there are animals that love common salt, while others want nothing to do with it. Every forester needs to put out salt in the winter, because certain animals need it. Farmers need salt for their sheep, which depend on it absolutely. This not only applies to animals, but in a certain way also to humans. There are tribes and peoples who don't appreciate common salt at all and have nothing to do with it, while others have fought huge historic battles in order to capture salt mines. Which animals require salt, and which peoples? It is the plant eaters who need salt, because in plants the quantity of potassium far exceeds that of sodium. Potassium is a constituent of solid substances and is found within the plant. As soon as we take in animal food, we don't need salt, because the animal as such

– the meat – is rich in sodium and magnesium. Under these circumstances we don't need additional salt, as excessive intake of salt can be poisonous. We will need to supplement salt intake again, however, as soon as we become plant eaters.

Obviously in certain illnesses we are overwhelmed with sodium, and so it is quite justified that Gerson lays emphasis on a sodium-free diet, and that he gives his patients nothing but a plant based diet. This forces the organism to break down the sodium in the body and to excrete it, and the organism becomes alkaline again. Now you should not imagine that this advice will lead to a crusade against common salt; it would be sectarian to believe that all illnesses can be healed in this way. Results have been experienced in certain cases of tuberculosis, such as lupus and similar conditions, while most other forms responded only slightly or not at all, and a cure was not achieved. In many cases salt is necessary.

When do people need salt (and lots of it) and when would one choose a salt-free diet? In cases of kidney disease, people are bloated; the bodily secretions have come to a standstill, because in a certain sense there is too much salt. Bloated, pale people need to be given very little salt; children with enlarged lymphatic glands need little salt, whereas thin children need to be given more salt. One thing that should not be used is iodised salt. It has a potential use in baths, but as a food supplement I regard it as completely misguided in all cases. In many places and in several cities I have witnessed children suffering severe thyroid disturbances as a result of taking iodised salt. Such minute doses can have unimaginably strong effects. People do not realise the explosive power contained in iodine. Tremendous forces are contained in the minutest quantities. Fundamentally iodine only exists in crystal form (as iodide salts), and when it is dissolved, it does not become liquid, but immediately turns into a gas; from this you can imagine the potentially destructive explosive power inherent within iodine. It is a substance to be treated with respect!

I have endeavoured to illustrate how different questions concerning patient diets may be approached.

In chronically ill patients nutrition must not be overlooked. The diet needs to play a supportive role to the medicines. This is the difference between an acute and a chronic illness. If you begin to live with the plant processes – with the flower, fruit and leaf processes; if with a loving heart you observe what takes place in a seed or a fruit, then through this observation you will see mighty powers at work: the sun, air, water, fire. You will observe how all the elements are at play within the plant, building up this being of the plant which is spread across the whole world. Then you begin to develop a sense – and this has been one of the aims of these lectures – for the healing qualities of food and nutrition.

Observation of the different kingdoms in nature needs to be cultivated. We need to differentiate between the meat of a cow and of a bird, how particular substances work in plants – for example, how spinach has a bitter taste because it contains so much iron, or how, since the tomato contains so much water and is red, certain processes are at work here, which are actually quite earthbound. Observe how a potato, which in the ground suddenly becomes a fruit, and yet is seemingly a root, stimulates different processes during digestion. Altogether the art of observation needs to be trained. It is only possible to give recipes when they are permeated with life, when one looks at nature in such a way that life itself reveals its essential qualities. I have tried to indicate the way you can look at foods within their context in the kingdoms of nature. It is of particular importance, to recognise how the entire activity of eating, digestion, metabolism, is not a material happening, but is altogether one of the most spiritual in our organism.

The thoughts that are being produced in the world nowadays – mostly accompanied by high-sounding feelings – are much more materialistic than everything that goes on in the process of human digestion. We therefore need to bow down before this process and open ourselves to receive a consciousness for the power of the force active in our metabolism. It is one of the mightiest and most powerful forces that hold sway in the human being.

Sitting down at table for a meal constitutes on the one hand the true meeting with nature and on the other with the forces of the universe. For if we sit at table to eat, we receive through the cosmic nutrition stream the cosmic forces which in our body are condensed and transubstantiated. On the other hand, eating gives us the possibility of de-materialising nature, thus liberating the forces living in her. Now we are able to observe these reciprocal processes where what comes from the spiritual world becomes earthly, while what comes from the earth becomes spiritual. Only when we once again look upon eating and food in this way will we arrive at a true and real culture of eating. The important thing is not – as is often attempted and longed for – that we as human beings return to simplicity. That is a misguided notion! It would mean denying our entire consciousness if we were to seek to go back to conditions that prevailed ten thousand years ago. We need to strive forwards and eventually attain a simplicity that is permeated with culture. One of the paths to achieving this – and I must honestly say that this would be particularly necessary in this locality – is the path of the right intake and preparation of food. Just this constitutes a path towards a spiritual enrichment of culture.

Basically we are constantly polluting our organism through food, and eating should really be a constant purification and healing of nature. Only when we are able to look upon it in this way in its full reality will we be able to recognise what it means to sit at table. In fact the greatest facts of earthly life and the most powerful events have taken place while sitting down and partaking of food. Just think of the Gospels. It is not for nothing that matters are described in this way, but in reality the most significant and purest impulses are intended to shine through the whole of earth existence and earth development. What keeps shining through the gospels as an image of the partaking of bread and wine, this sacramental eating process needs to become an experience for us again.

These considerations have been offered in the hope that they will be taken up by you all on a practical level.

The Cultural Impulse
of Agriculture

*Three lectures on milk and nutrition at Heathcot House,
Aberdeen October 15 to 18, 1943*

Auch
ein
Tischgebet.

Es schwimmen die Fische in des Meeres Grund.
Es leuchtet ihr Wesen im Spiel der Wellen.
Und wandelt die Wärme im Lichte des Äthers.

So wandelt sich Nahrung im Menschen-Innern.
So leuchtet Substanz auf durch Menschenkraft.
So wiegt sich der Mensch im Arme der Gottheit.

———

✣

beendet
20. IX. 1943

Another Table Grace

The fish swim in the depth of the sea.
Their being shines in the play of the waves.
And transforms the warmth in the light of the ether.

Thus is transformed the food in the body of man.
Thus substance lights up through human forces.
Thus is man cradled in the arms of the Godhead.

Completed September 20, 1943, from one of Karl König's notebooks

1 Milk and Blood

Lecture 1, Friday morning, October 15, 1943

I have been asked to address the subject of food, including nutrition and digestion. In three lectures it is almost impossible to do justice to this complex and very important subject. Even if there were the possibility of speaking for two or three months, we could not fully cover this subject for the simple reason that not enough is known about food, about nutrition, about digestion and about the whole realm of human metabolism. It is especially apparent to those doctors who have started to study anthroposophical medicine that they are only at the very beginning, so please do not expect too much from me, because what I am able to bring can amount at most to a few fundamental and perhaps startling facts.

A start has to be made, however, and so I venture to address you in this conference, even if it is only to make a beginning. Hundreds of years of research lie ahead before we will understand the secret and the hidden riddle of nutrition, digestion and metabolism. To begin with I will attempt to convey to you how anthroposophy has taught us to see phenomena. Rudolf Steiner once expressed himself to medical doctors in a very candid way:

> Your task is to study all that science has produced in our time, all that science has brought to light. The greatest inspirations can be derived from studying an ordinary book on physiology or anatomy, because science has

121

gathered together all the phenomena you need to know, science has brought together all these facts, and this is a wonderful achievement.[1]

What we have to do is integrate this multitude of fragmentary facts. By providing them, science has actually placed the tools into our hands, but the new task is to gather them all together and allow a new interpretation of the human being, of the cosmic world and everything around us to arise from them. Anthroposophy opens up for us this world of possibility. The tools are so widely scattered that it is absolutely impossible for any single human being to study them all. Even a whole lifetime would not suffice; our spiritual power is anyway too limited, but perhaps a few facts and points of view will lead you to appreciate how a meaningful collaboration between physicians and farmers could commence anew, illumined by what anthroposophy can bring to the facts provided by science.

If nowadays for instance you study a book on nutrition written by a doctor or scientist – usually by a scientist (doctors are less able to write such books because they still retain some understanding of the human being) – you will find a vast list of facts and figures presented, yet they don't really lead to any significant conclusion; they merely confirm the results of experiments and are not really of any practical use.

If you study a current [1943] textbook on the function of the intestinal tract, on the physiology of digestion, you will find that digestion is still regarded as a process that exists in order to produce heat and substance for the human or animal organism. Not so very long ago – as a matter of fact it is even the case today – in most books on the physiology of nutrition, the human organism, is considered to be nothing but a kind of stove, with food as the fuel that keeps the stove going. Meanwhile, science has recognised a complication, namely that the fuel and the stove must be related to each other in some peculiar way, because the fuel is able to build up the stove, and the stove, which is destroying the fuel, is built up by this same destructive process.

Let me describe how, for instance, butter, milk and meat change inside our digestive tract, what processes these foodstuffs have to go through, and how they eventually appear somewhere else in the organism in a modified condition.

I have studied many books on this question, but the more one reads about it, the more obvious it becomes just how little these facts of digestion are as yet actually understood. For instance, it is not known (and I do not mean only within the scientific hierarchy, I mean by all of us) how the proteins in meat are metabolised, and how they appear later on beyond the intestinal wall. The way they pass through our intestine and are transformed there, is mere conjecture rather than certain knowledge. So far it has it has not been possible to observe the basic facts. It is assumed that food is split up chemically, that it is split up physically, and is then changed into very simple substances; these go through the intestinal wall, are taken up by the lymph and enter the bloodstream. This is one possible hypothesis, but I do not believe that this is an adequate explanation. And no scientist is in a position to disprove it because he is not able to prove the contrary on the basis of experimental facts – and so one must try and understand the whole question from a different premise, starting with some facts which I think are very familiar to you.

I shall not begin with the process of digestion, but with a description of milk; I would like you to follow me as a physician in considering this substance, as familiar as it may to be to all of you as farmers.

As doctors, we too ought to be very interested in the question of what milk is – after all it is not only produced by cows, but by many other animals, including humans, to feed their offspring. Our mothers create milk, and with regard to the human being, milk is the only food that the human being is able to produce. All other foods are created by Mother Nature, by Mother Earth. Milk is produced by human beings during a certain period of time, namely when a portion of humanity enters the state of motherhood. Suddenly, after the woman has given birth to her baby, she comes into a condition in which the whole of nature seems to create a substance, milk, within the human body.

Throughout the year, food is produced outside the human body, but one particular food – milk – is produced by the human being during a certain period of life. Milk is one of the most important foodstuffs we have. Without our mothers' milk we would hardly be able to live. Humans share this great possibility of producing milk with many other beings, with all mammals, which are also able to produce milk and so to feed their newborn offspring.

Consider what it means that we as members of the human kingdom are able to produce food in the form of milk. It means that during the production of milk, the human being – or perhaps I should say, the woman – enters the realm of Nature with her whole being. The woman stands within the realm of Nature as a food-producing creature. But this food is produced specifically for her own baby to whom she has given birth.

Now you all know that milk is a white opaque fluid that tastes slightly sweet and contains a wide range of different substances. We know that it contains sugar, protein and certain fatty substances, but that it also contains many minerals, for instance manganese, copper, iron, magnesium, potassium, calcium and so on. Virtually the whole realm of substances appears within milk. You can find the whole of Nature gathered together in one spot, within a single substance.

Milk is a colloidal fluid with a slightly sweet taste, originating, as it were, from the mammary glands, where it is produced. But in reality these glands, through the sacrifice of their own tissue, create or produce milk. The production of milk does not merely involve the creation of this fluid. It represents, so to speak, a process of self-sacrifice of the milk glands, since milk is built up by the destruction of all the cells of the tubules of the milk glands. Milk represents, if you will, the outcome of the sacrifice of a specific glandular tissue in the human or animal organism.

When, as a doctor, you have the opportunity of accompanying a pregnant woman and observe those wonderful changes that the whole organism undergoes, you will notice that as the breasts are growing, there is a considerable increase in their blood supply. Hundreds of new blood vessels develop around the milk glands within the breasts. Observation of this awakens in us the realisation that blood is not merely necessary for the production of milk, but that blood is, so to speak, the very mother-substance out of which milk is produced. In this connection I recently came across a paper containing the following statement:

> A given amount of blood supply is needed to produce a given amount of milk; in fact four times as much blood is needed for the production of a given amount of milk.[2]

This means that four units of blood are needed for the breast to produce one unit of milk. This particular relationship between blood and milk is reminiscent of another relationship manifesting the same ratio, namely the rhythm between the pulse and the breathing process. For each breath of inhalation and exhalation we have four pulse beats. This leads us to the realisation that the secretion of milk can be related to the breathing process. I would like you first of all to bear this thought in mind before pursuing our understanding of the substance of milk from a different direction.

Yesterday evening Dr Lehrs reminded us of Luke Howard's beautiful words from his book about the forms of clouds.[3] We are invited to observe and learn once again to understand the countenance of the atmosphere, and everything going on in it. Yet despite the lapse of time we still have not regained the possibility of reading the countenance of the atmosphere surrounding us. We have yet to relearn what Luke Howard tried to discern in studying cloud formations. Goethe made a similar attempt. In times gone by, people were not only able to read the countenance of the atmosphere, they were able to read what lay behind its countenance; what made this countenance appear as it did; what, so to speak, created the features of the clouds, the rain and thunder storms and everything surrounding the being of the earth.

It is now about twenty years since Rudolf Steiner gave a lecture describing the atmosphere as it was in the Lemurian Age and the Atlantean Epoch of earth evolution.[4] I think that farmers would benefit from reading and re-reading this lecture. Without going into details, this lecture reveals the whole secret of the two substances of calcium and silica that are so very important both to farmers and doctors.

I would like to relate what Rudolf Steiner said there about the early Lemurian epoch in a few words. He describes how the whole atmosphere in the early Lemurian epoch was nothing but a huge cloud of protein. If a modern chemist were to speak about this protein, he would not be able to speak about it in terms of carbon, nitrogen, hydrogen or oxygen for the simple reason that these substances did not exist at that time. But protein did exist, and the whole atmosphere was filled with this cloud of protein, and this protein was warmed through by life. There were no elements – no carbon, nitrogen, oxygen, sulphur and phosphorus; they simply did not exist. How are we to understand this – one of Rudolf Steiner's most significant revelations? The basic elements did not gradually link together in the distant past, and in so doing create more and more complicated molecules, from which eventually, by a particularly fortuitous conglomeration, the first molecule was created, out of which the whole world of life gradually evolved. Although this is what science proclaims today, it is simply not true.

Protoplasm existed first of all. The whole atmosphere was filled with a substance that was not a complicated one, but a simple one. Out of this very simple substance the complexity of elements as we know them gradually separated out. The original unit was just simple protoplasm, filling the atmosphere of earliest earth existence.

In the early Lemurian period, the whole atmosphere of the

earth was a big cloud of protoplasm, warmed through by life, which was cosmic life. From the cosmos, like rain, silica was dripping in; not silica that was hard like granite, but constituted more like wax. This was dripping down. There was light, and this light was reflected by the silica wax; and with the light 'archetypal cosmic images' were streaming down into the atmosphere – and these archetypal images constituted the first plants. They were not like our plants, with a definite form and shape – these plants were more like coloured movements, appearing and disappearing. The whole earth was still within the process of creation, nothing attained permanence – but everything was continuously being created and dissolved again.

Rudolf Steiner revealed that it was not only this wax-like form of silica that dripped down from the cosmos into this albuminous atmosphere of the earth. Calcium or lime too rained down form the cosmic surroundings into the earth. And then he described a very important phenomenon:

> As the rain is now falling down onto the earth and rising
> up again, so during the Lemurian epoch, lime was raining
> downwards and evaporating upwards. There was a raining
> down of lime substance descending and then rising up, a
> real stream of lime from the cosmic world down to the
> earth, and from the earth up into the cosmos.[5]

During this time, within this atmosphere of protein, other things were taking place. Parts of the albumin coagulated, giving rise to the first rather primitive animals. The lime then penetrated these clotted protein coagulations constituting these first and primitive animals, giving rise to the first very primitive cartilaginous formations. These animals had the ability to extend a limb and retract it again; however, they did not yet have a fixed and defined shape. It is a Philistine attitude to assume that the animals around us are the perfect ones. They are sclerotic beings because they have a defined form. Nothing more can be done with such animals. But these early Lemurian prototypes were able to adapt themselves to the atmospheric conditions, where the calcium or lime rain was able to stream in and out: these were the true animals.

In this picture of how the atmosphere of the early beginnings of our earth was built up, I have actually described something that can still be observed today, namely the substance milk. Were we to observe a glass of milk for 24 hours, we would be able to follow what once upon a time had taken place in the early Lemurian epoch. What had once been the atmosphere – the early cloud – albeit a great deal smaller, is still here. And in milk you have the real image of everything that had once existed in the creation of the world. This is why at the beginning of life we have to feed our babies with milk; we cannot feed them anything else, because thereby they partake in creation; moreover, they not only renew the body, but something else as well.

If you read books by Paracelsus, you may come across certain passages where he speaks about milk. He always refers to milk by a very funny name: he calls it the 'Good Mummy' [*die gute Mumie*]. Over against this 'Good Mummy' he says there is another mummy, the 'Bad Mummy,' of which every farmer and doctor should be aware. This 'Bad Mummy' is contained in urine, he says. What does this mean? We cannot really understand this unless we study what science has brought to light – and it is very necessary to study these facts. This is the point where the birth takes place; we know that it takes ten [lunar] months, or 280 days, for the baby to be fully formed, and now let us study for how long the milk production of the mother goes on:

280 days	*birth*	
		280 days

It is also exactly ten months, or 280 days. It is a singular fact that the length of time it takes for a baby to be fully formed is the same as the length of time the mother's breasts have the power to produce milk. And if you read the book on physiology by C.G. Carus, a contemporary of Goethe's, he says that you can only understand the production of milk in a woman if you grasp the fact that after the birth all the forces that have created the embryo rise up into the breasts, where they then create the milk.[6] This means that all the embryonic forces that were bestowed on the mother by the cosmos now stream into the breast and build up the milk. When the baby drinks milk, it is drinking the 'Good Mummy' – the cosmic mother. All the cosmic forces that have created the baby now stream into the mother, and this is what the baby is drinking.

If you were able to follow the process the milk creates in the baby, and listened very carefully when the milk arrived in the baby's stomach and intestine, you might sometimes be able to hear that the milk talks. And the milk says, 'Come, come, come.' It calls down the spiritual being of the baby. Only milk is able to do this so gently and kindly that the soul of the baby responds and grows into the baby during these nine or ten months of breast-feeding.

I do not mean to say that one should breastfeed the baby entirely and exclusively up to the ninth month. At six months one should start giving some other food, and steadily increase this until the child is finally weaned by nine months. Only in certain tribal societies are children breastfed up to the age of three years. This would not be conducive to producing children with the alert minds required by modern conditions of life.

We had a boy in our schools who was very slow in his whole development and I was able to trace this back to the fact that he had been breastfed for too long. Animals deprived of mother's milk suffer in their physical development but not otherwise. In human beings the effects are seen in psychological development.

When babies do not get their mother's milk, but cow's milk or other milk, the soul is not called down gently, but pulled down too vigorously. The forces entering the body are not able to settle down properly, making the baby thin and weak.

I am now not going to speak about human milk and cow's milk, but I would like to say something about the substances in milk so that you can see how similar milk is to blood. Blood is red and milk is white, but both are opaque. The reason for this is their colloidal state. All the blood cells are suspended in the blood serum, and all the tiny fat globules are suspended in the milk.

If you were to remove all the blood corpuscles, you would have blood serum. If you take all the fat globules out of the milk, you have a serum too. If you study both serums, you will find that they are very similar; they consist of the same substances. Both serums contain a protein – in milk it is caseinogen, in blood it is fibrinogen. Fibrinogen causes blood to clot. Caseinogen causes milk to curdle. You then find in blood a certain amount of globulins and albumins, and the same globulins and albumins are found in milk serum.

What does all this signify? I would say that the only difference between blood and milk lies in the nature of these tiny particles that make blood and milk opaque. The blood corpuscles, particularly the red corpuscles in the blood, and the fat globules in milk are the same. From a biological point of view they are really the same, for in milk a state is reached which can only be found in the earliest stages of human embryological development.

In a human embryo at about 14, 15, 16 days after fertilisation, the yolk-sac is built up, and within the yolk-sac you find the yolk substance, which is not very well researched, because not many young embryos are available. The yolk sac is there, and inside this yolk sac there is a beautiful golden fluid, which is called the yolk. If it is exposed to light, this fatty yolk substance is destroyed. The human embryo is only nourished by this for a very short time. The first rudiments of blood and blood vessels are formed in the yolk sac.

In milk the yolk appears too, this time not before, but after embryonic development. It appears in such a way that it is newly created out of the blood – and you should contemplate the following cycle. In the Lemurian epoch there was milk, and we were all living as spiritual beings in this milky condition, side by side with the animals and plants, which were just beginning to become physical. We were all living inside this 'cosmic milk'. Then we came closer and closer to earthly life; we incarnated more and more, and, so to speak, as a self-defence against this milk of the gods, we created our own *personal milk*. And this *personal milk* – this sinful milk, which has to be redeemed – is our blood.

Nature again and again redeems this blood at certain moments by re-creating in the mother's breasts the real milk, which corresponds to the cosmic milk of the Lemurian epoch.

Now study the cloud formations, study cirrus, cumulus, stratus and nimbus, and study the milk in your bottles. You will find that the cirrus clouds correspond to the skin formed by milk, and cumulus is the fat that turns into butter. Stratus is nothing but the caseinogen, and nimbus is the whey. You will have to look at the clouds to see whether your milk will keep – whether it will be colonised by bacteria or not.

This is a way of learning again how to see substance, because milk does not consist of carbon, hydrogen, oxygen and so on. Milk consists of one thing only, and that is – *milk*. But to study milk does not mean to study all the constituent parts. To study milk means to study cheese, butter, whey, milking, atmospheric influences and so on; only then will you be able to understand milk.

One should write a song about milk, because you cannot imagine what a beautiful substance it is. It is really the song of the whole creation. It is not the minerals, salts, fats and other constituents which make the baby grow better when it is breastfed – the whole creation is streaming into the baby's body in the milk, and this makes the baby grow.

131

Let me read to you what a modern scientist has to say in a book on human physiology:

> We know very little about the mechanism of milk secretion. It seems impossible at present to explain the very close adaptation between the secretory cells and the needs of the infant or young animal.[7]

To become consciously aware of these needs again may help the farmer. There is an old tale told by the farmers of Australia. They say that the young kangaroos do not come out of the womb, but that they bud on the teats of their mothers. Scientists were astonished at this idea and went to investigate these very interesting animals, and discovered the following: the kangaroos produce the embryos within the womb, where they grow only to about an inch in size. When they are born, the mother goes down with her lips, takes them up and puts them into her pouch, and in this pouch she presses the lips of the little ones onto the teats. The lips are the biggest organs of these embryos. The lips then grow around the teats and form a kind of placenta. For six months the embryos hang suspended to the teats whilst they grow to maturity. And what does the milk do? Imagine the lips – and milk continually dripping down from the teats into the mouths of the babies. These drops of milk form a kind of living umbilical cord between mother and baby.

This is what a doctor should know, but perhaps a farmer may contemplate such things too.

Discussion

Question: If the baby dies, what can one do for the mother?
Karl König: It is possible to give a certain medicine to lead the milk-producing process outwards via the kidneys. There are medicinal herbs that can do this.

An unrecorded question was asked.
Karl König: Blood contains iron, milk contains magnesium. Magnesium is the cosmic counterpart of iron. It is significant that pure magnesium is only found in meteors. It is not found in the earth except where meteors have fallen.

Question: What happens when milk is pasteurised?
Karl König: You remove the 'Good Mummy' form the cow's milk when you pasteurise it; it is then replaced by the 'Bad Mummy.'

The cow is a special animal within creation. All measures and proportions of the cosmos are the same in the cow. When you drink the etheric forms of the cow's milk you drink the power of the cosmos. When you pasteurise milk, you destroy these forces.

Question: Does freezing harm milk?
Karl König: Yes, I am sure it does. You destroy the form of the etheric forces. The fat is then surrounded by caseinogen, and the whole composition of the milk altered.

An unrecorded question was asked.
Karl König: A milk diet is good for ulcers.

Questions were asked about the use of mistletoe, and about plant/vegetable milk as compared to animal milk.
Karl König: We use mistletoe as a treatment for cancer. All the

plant milks have a certain connection with animal milk – but they act more through the liver. The liver is the only place where fibrinogen and caseinogen are produced.

A question was asked about the use of iodine to stimulate milk production in cows.

Karl König: Milk was once deprived of iodine. Feeding cows thyroid preparations will enhance milk production for a certain time – and then the cow will die. What iodine does in the short term, oil cakes do in the longer term. Salt licks are effective because they contain iodine.

Lord Glentanar: I can speak from personal experience on this subject, as I am guilty of using such things. I used to win cups for high milk yields for many years, but eventually all my cows died.

There followed a discussion about the lack of iodine in South America and the consequences of this for cows and breeding. Then there was a question about appropriate feed for breeding stock.

Mr Duffy: At the present time [during the second World War] it is difficult to feed appropriately, as all grain is requisitioned by the government, but as much as possible should be retained, even if it is only the chaff from the wheat for the breeding animals. One solution would be to grow a mixture of oats, barley and peas. It is permitted to feed this to cattle. Silage in large quantities is detrimental. Silage could be reserved for fattening up bullocks, for example.

Karl König: Nowadays we keep our animals in dark stables and give them feed that has been kept in the dark (silage). Thereby we deprive the cows of the forces of light.

Mr Duffy: One of the most amazing medicines is Silica D7. When I say that we have never lost a cow, I do not say that we have never been in danger of losing one, but through the use of the biological medicines we have been able to save them. These preparations are now available from the Present Age Company, as Weleda has stopped producing them due to difficulties caused by the war.

2 Faeces and the Brain

Lecture 2, Friday evening, October 15, 1943

This morning we have tried to develop an understanding of the nature of milk. I hope you were able to experience how in contemplating an archetypal phenomenon like milk we are lead not only to an understanding of nature, but also into the realm of evolution, into the very creation of earth and man. By simply tracing the facts and then trying to interpret them, we were really able to unfold an understanding, which I, at least, find very meaningful.

I have chosen the subject of milk this morning because it is a biological substance with which you as farmers are familiar. Tonight I will continue to speak about this substance, but from a different angle. It will become clear as I speak about digestion that the nature of milk is being addressed from a different point of view.

Most of you will be familiar with the last lecture of Rudolf Steiner's Agriculture Course, held in 1924. In this eighth lecture Rudolf Steiner spoke – I believe for the first time – about the human brain. He reveals the existence of a very important connection, or rather, a profound relationship between the brain on the one hand and dung or faeces on the other. This is indeed a startling revelation; even more startling is that Rudolf Steiner went on to say that the brain is essentially to be understood as a kind of dung formation.

Now you may well ask, what does this mean? It is possible

gradually to arrive at an understanding of the fact that the brain can indeed be seen as a kind of dung formation – and to appreciate that this understanding may benefit my work as a physician, in relation to both human beings and animals.

Long before giving these lectures to farmers, Rudolf Steiner had given a series of medical lectures to doctors. There he revealed another startling fact, which I think has to be linked with what he indicated in the Agriculture Course.

> The more the forebrain develops in the course of animal evolution, eventually assuming the form it has in the human being, the more the intestines develop in the direction that leads to storing the remains of food. There is an intimate connection between the formation of intestines and the formation of the brain; if the colon and the appendix had not appeared in the course of the evolution of animals, physical human beings who can think would also ultimately not have been able to appear, because humans have brains at the expense – at the very pronounced expense – of their intestinal organs.
>
> The intestinal organs are the faithful obverse of the structures in the brain.[1]

I was particularly struck by this remark. I first read it in 1926 or 1927, and even then I wondered whether it might be possible to discover facts that might substantiate this statement. A year later I came across a paper published in 1927 in the *Archiv für Anatomie,* dealing with the connection between the intestinal and the cerebral structure in humans and animals. This paper also contains a description of the astonishing correspondence between brain and intestine. It was written by a well-known professor of anatomy, a scientist, who was simply studying facts, and basing his conclusions on these facts rather than on any hypothesis, be it Darwinian or any other. It is summed up in the concluding passages, where he wrote:

There exists a strange kind of parallelism between the number of intestinal convolutions and the number of cerebral convolutions. It is an incontestable fact that the bigger the number of intestinal convolutions, the more convolutions there are on the surface of the brain. There is no doubt that from Didelphys up to humans, the cerebral cortex grows ever more complex. But it has not been possible to trace any phylogenetic development.[2]

What he is drawing attention to is that although it has not been possible to correlate the brains of different vertebrates with the tree of evolution, in every species the number of convolutions in the intestine correspond to the number of convolutions in the brain. If this is found to be the case in so many vertebrates, there must be a reason for it.

Let us take this fact and relate it to Rudolf Steiner's remark. They both appear to refer to the relationship between brain and dung; the function of the intestine and the convolutions of the brain are in a kind of equilibrium with each other. What could this mean? If we turn to human physiology and study the faeces, study what faeces are made of, where they come from, we will discover even more interesting and starling facts; and the more we study them, the more startling these facts become. Neither laymen nor doctors are aware of them – but these facts should become generally known and familiar to all.

Faeces have little to do with the intake of food, because whether we eat or starve makes comparatively little difference to the content and amount of faeces. A person starving for ten, twelve, fourteen or sixteen days does not produce much less faeces every day to the person who is eating. This is a startling fact. The food is completely broken down, and therefore there are hardly any nutrients in faeces from healthy people. Students are never asked any questions about faeces in examinations. You do not study the subject either as a student or as a doctor. But you can read about it in Starling's *Principles of Human Physiology*. Starling writes:

> In humans or carnivores, the absorption of the constituents of a meal is practically complete by the time the food has arrived at the lower end of the ileum. The faeces are in the main not derived from the food, but are produced almost entirely in the alimentary canal itself. This is shown by the fact that on analysing the faeces, no soluble carbohydrates or proteins, albumoses, peptones or amino acids are found. After a meal of meat, microscopical examination of the faeces reveals no trace of striated muscle fibres. Moreover, in a state of complete starvation, animals form faeces that do not differ in composition from faeces formed after feeding, though the amount is smaller.

In one experiment, Johann Hermann (1738–1800) isolated a loop of gut, joining its ends together so that a continuous ring was formed. After some weeks, the isolated loop was found to contain a semi-solid material similar to faeces. This is a very important experiment. Here I will give you the proportions of the constituents of faeces:

- Water 65–67%
- Nitrogen 5–9%
- Ether Extract 12–18% (used to determine the fat content)
- Ash 11–22%

Starling writes: 'The material basis of faeces seems to be largely inspissated mucus, bile and other secretions, desquamated epithelial cells form the intestinal wall, and bacteria, of which countless numbers of chiefly dead [ones] are present.'

The production of dung in the human and animal body has very little to do with consumed food. Of course, if indigestible material enters the gut, it certainly goes into the faeces, for instance, bones, cellulose, etc. are excreted with the faeces. This material is something that is found there too, but it constitutes only a minor part of the faeces.[3] Essentially, the faeces are not formed by food, but are a product of the intestinal mucosa, of the whole gut. But what does this intestinal mucosa consist of? When you study the hundreds of experiments that have been done with regard to digestion and metabolism, you will find that we are only able to digest food because the intestine secretes a tremendous quantity of intestinal juices. These are produced by the mouth, in the stomach, in the duodenum and in the small intestine, as well as in the large intestine. Throughout the entire intestinal tract there are millions of minute glands, and these tiny glands start to secrete this intestinal juice immediately after the intake of food.[4]

Now you must imagine that the moment you take in food, when you are hungry, or even when you only see a nicely laid table, when you smell something appetising, the whole of the intestinal tract starts to secrete this juice. This juice is one of the most important secretions our body produces. Only through the production of this juice is digestion possible. But what is the real meaning of the word 'to digest'? What is actually done to the food when we digest? If you take milk, for instance, but instead of drinking it, you inject it directly into the bloodstream – what happens? The recipient will start to develop a very high temperature. Milk can even be used in this way to raise temperatures.

The moment we inject milk directly into the bloodstream, we ourselves as a biological entity have to fight the other biological entity that has been introduced. We start to fight it rather vigorously, and a symptom of this is the raised temperature. Afterwards our own biological entity returns to normal. It is important to realise that any kind of food we ingest is poison to the human biological entity. It is poison because it is a foreign substance, and digestion implies the destruction of what is of an alien nature to ourselves. We have to break down these foreign substances to single units, both chemically and physically, and only after they have nearly been destroyed are we fully ourselves again. You know how difficult it is to think clearly after a heavy meal. This is merely the expression of the fact that in digestion we are engaged in a fight against alien substance, the food, and after ingesting a heavy meal, for instance, we have little possibility of solving a difficult problem.

Our knowledge must expand to be able to understand that digestion is a battle against alien entities, whether these are cabbages, pork or sugar – they are all alien to us. This battle is fought by the intestinal juices, and these intestinal juices are the means by which our biological entity destroys the alien foodstuffs.

What does this signify? Imagine this to be our mouth, and here we take in the food, which gradually descends more and more, arriving eventually at the walls of the small intestine.

As soon as we take in food we start to produce intestinal juices; they are already produced in our mouth through the

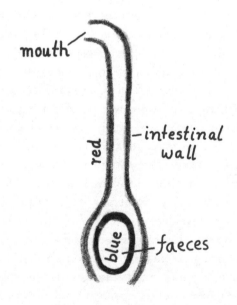

salivary glands, then in the stomach, then in the duodenum and then in the small intestine. Faeces comprise the product of the different juices of the intestinal tract. Wherever it may originate, this juice, whether from the intestinal wall, the pancreas or the liver, most of what is contained in this juice is then excreted. It is very important to realise this, to accustom oneself to the idea that faeces are essentially the product of the intestinal juices and not of the food itself.

Let us now consider another of Rudolf Steiner's statements. He spoke in a clear way about the structure of the brain – describing it as the only organ in the body that, with regard to its substance, is really built up by the food that is ingested.[5] Everything else, muscles, bones, all the organs, are not built up by the substances we eat as food. Only one organ is able to utilise these substances, and that is the brain. I will indicate this in the following drawing: here we have the food, represented by a blue line and forming the brain. On the one side we have the intake

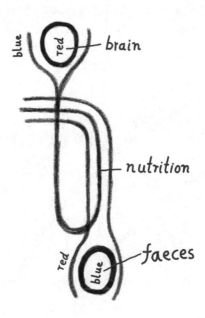

141

of substances, from which something precipitates, namely the brain. The faeces resulting from our food constitute the brain. As a mirror image of this process, the actual faeces are formed from the intestinal juice through a process of precipitation.

It would appear that these two substances, the brain and the faeces, must be somehow connected. Is it possible to conceive how this stream of food reaches the brain? I do not think that anybody really knows, although both science and anthroposophy have constructed some models. One may conclude from experiments that the wall of the intestinal tract, of the small as well as of the large intestine, constitutes a threshold through which nothing can pass, from inside out (red arrow). When the intestine is in a healthy condition, it does not seem possible for any kind of substance to pass through the intestinal wall. When you study the histological structure of the intestinal wall, you find thousands and thousands of little villi. These tiny villi reach into the inside of the intestine. Today science holds the following view: the food which is taken in, which is broken down and destroyed by the intestinal juice (by the juice produced by the millions of intestinal glands), is absorbed through the action of the villi, passes through the intestinal wall and enters the lymph vessels.

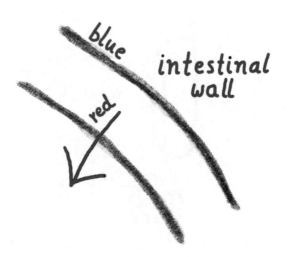

A certain portion of it eventually does reach the bloodstream via the lymph stream. (The food inside the intestinal wall is called chyme, and beyond the intestinal wall it is called chyle.)

The villi float in the intestinal juice, mingled and mixed with all the substances into which the food has been transformed. What do the villi actually do? They are considered to be performing a kind of sucking process, sucking up the chime. Now bring to mind a natural process: a baby sucking at the mother's breast, or a calf at the udder of a cow. The wall of the intestine is like thousands or millions of little udders. Does the udder now take something from the calf, or the calf from the udder? The conception of science today in regard to these intestinal villi is as if we were to say that the udder is sucking from the calf! This certainly does not happen. But the question remains: by what means is the food extracted from the intestine? How is it possible for food that is taken in to pass through the intestinal wall, or does it perhaps not pass through the intestinal wall at all?

Analysis of the lymph behind the intestinal walls or of the bloodstream after the intake of a meal does not reveal the presence of proteins. There is no increase in proteins, no increase in sugars, no increase in carbohydrates in the lymph and bloodstream around the intestinal wall. This can be verified in humans as well as in animals. Only one substance is found there in increased quantities, and that is fat. There are no proteins or carbohydrates; yet one has found *no* fatty globules in these villi. Although the intestinal wall has been studied microscopically hundreds and thousands of times, never has any drop of fat been found; yet *behind* it there was fat and in front of it there was fat as well as other substances.[6] This seems to suggest that substances are being *newly created*.

Now if one is not a professor of physiology, but has retained some common sense, it might occur to ask the question, how did the fat get form the one side to the other? Might there be a pathway we still do not know of, that we still cannot conceive? There must be a form of transport at work, which I can only conceive of in the following way: *matter is entirely dissolved inside the intestinal tract, and is newly re-created on the other side of the intestinal tract,* and thus the intestinal wall indeed constitutes a real wall. There is no possible means of transport in three-dimensional space; yet a way of transport is certainly conceivable in other dimensions.

Might one imagine that each substance – sugar, carbohydrates, and so on, is taken up into an etheric condition, and is precipitated on the other side in a physical condition? When we take in carbon, we have to destroy the living substance of the carbon. Eating it means dissolving it into a very simple substance. We now have to take hold of this substance again and fill it with our own living etheric body, and this process takes place through *raising the substance up* on the one hand, and lowering it on the other side of the intestinal wall. You have to climb over a wall to understand what happens to the food between the inside and the outside the intestine. That the food has to traverse a wall means *to change from a physical state into an etheric state and then down to a physical state again.*

Beyond the intestinal wall, the lymph-stream is filled again with fatty substances, with proteins and minerals, which rise up to feed the brain; they do not feed anything else in the body. Our brain is formed out of the substance that has become our own substance just because it is beyond the intestine. This now constitutes the substance of our own human biological entity.

This morning I spoke to you about the nature of milk; two products are derived from milk: the one is butter, the other cheese. I don't plan to tell you anything about the making of butter or cheese. You certainly know much more about this than I do. But let us consider cheese as a biological entity. What is it? When you eat butter and when you eat cheese you have two quite different sensations. You have two quite different experiences, and yet both substances are derived from milk. On the one hand through a more or less quiet process the fatty substances of the milk gather together and clot through a certain rhythmical movement applied to it; and at the end we have butter, and out flows the 'serum' of the milk. Butter is the compound of all those fat globules that make milk into an opaque liquid; the serum runs out.

With cheese it is different. To make cheese you have to apply a substance that derives from the stomach of an animal – rennet. You have to apply something that is part of the intestinal juice. This special component of the intestinal juice works upon certain proteins, and the caseins clump together; this process, which the casein undergoes, takes the particles of fat along with it, and so cheese is obtained, containing more or less fat. The casein in milk as a substance corresponds to fibrinogen in blood. And this caseinogen substance is obtained from milk by applying to it a component of intestinal juice.

In butter we have a substance obtained through a quiet and rhythmical process, but cheese is something that goes through a process like digestion in the intestine. There are certain cheeses in which you can even smell this connection. Do not think that I want to denigrate cheese. I like it very much, but one cannot deny the similarity.

Now I am going to make a proposition, which I believe to be true, but please simply take it as a hypothesis. The food we take in mixes and mingles with the juice of the intestinal tract. If you can see this intestinal mixture and touch it with your hands you feel that this is milk, which is continually being created when the food substances derived from nature and human intestinal juices mix together. Two worlds are being mixed: the human world through the juices of the intestinal tract, and the food taken from the realm of nature. This milk within our own body undergoes the same two processes that occur when we make butter and cheese out of ordinary milk.

Our brain consists of nothing but fatty substances. I can remember (I do not know whether it is the same in this country), many years ago, when I was still a boy, the farmers used to bring their butter to Vienna, and each piece was shaped like a

walnut, which looked wonderful. It was in the form of a walnut!
I can still see it in my mind's eye, and I can still remember what
I felt when I saw this butter. I had the same feeling later when
reading in Strindberg's *Blaubuch* about the relationship between
the walnut and the brain, which Strindberg was able to describe
very intimately. The formation of the brain as Rudolf Steiner
described it, may be likened to butter made from the mixture
of intestinal juice and food, and faeces are essentially a form of
cheese. We may have tasted a wonderful cheese, in which we
could smell this connection between faeces and cheese, yet it
tasted very good. When we study these things from the point
of view of taste and smell, and note the sensation, we will come
to understand them. We don't only have milk produced in the
breasts, we have milk produced in the small intestine; this milk
goes through a further process, and you will understand why
Rudolf Steiner said that the brain is a kind of faeces in which the
whole process has not come to an end. Cheese and butter, faeces
and brain, they both originate in this nutritional stream. We will
consider the stream of cosmic nutrition in the third lecture.

3 The Rain of Cosmic Nutrition

Lecture 3, Sunday afternoon, October 17, 1943

On Friday evening I made an attempt (I hope not completely unsuccessfully) to speak about the nutritional stream. I tried to show that one has to consider the intestinal wall – particularly in humans, but not so completely in animals – as a real threshold; and that hardly any food, whether destroyed or not, passes through this intestinal wall. The whole process of digestion and metabolism can be thought of in such a way that on the one side food is broken down more or less completely, and on the other side, beyond the intestinal wall, the food is rebuilt, but rebuilt from a quite different source: from etheric forces it is rebuilt right down into physical substance.

I also tried to show that faeces on the one side, and the brain on the other, result from this whole process. I will repeat the drawings that I made as a reminder of this.

Here is the nutrition stream, which is dissolved into the milk of digestion, and beyond the intestinal wall is the [blue] substance stream of nutrition, to be built up into the fatty substances which nourish the brain. We spoke about gastric and intestinal juice, and how this juice is really breaking down all the fatty and other substances, and how, together with the broken down and dissolved food it forms this intestinal milk, the milk of nutrition [red, downward]. The result – the physical result of the

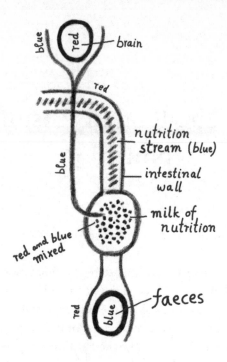

intestinal juice – is the faeces, which I compared to cheese made from the milk of nutrition. On the other hand, I compared the brain to the 'butter' from this milk of nutrition. And then a discussion began, and we could see how difficult it is to grasp these concepts, to begin to understand that the faeces have little to do with the intake of food, but that the brain has a lot to do with the actual, physical intake of food. Faeces are largely the residue of this gastric and intestinal juice, there being hardly any other sources for them.

This leads to the question, from where does this special and unique intestinal juice originate? We know that the intestinal juice is secreted by the glands lining the whole wall of the large and small intestine, but what causes this juice to flow? Why does it flow? Is there anything else known about this juice?

Here I have to mention the name of a great scientist, who really first alerted the stubborn heads of physiologists to the fact that digestion and metabolism are much more closely connected with the whole of the human being than anybody in the world of science had previously imagined. I am referring to the Russian physiologist Ivan Petrovich Pavlov. He died a very old man in 1936. In the first part of his life he undertook thousands of the most ingenious experiments to show that the flow of the intestinal and gastric juices is not only something which takes place like any other reaction in the body, but that this flow of the intestinal juice is brought about even in the absence of food. By his experiments Professor Pavlov was able show that an amazing intelligence and wisdom is at work in our body, because these gastric and intestinal juices, and even the secretions of the salivary glands, exactly match the kind of food we eat, be it meat, sweet or savoury. The composition of the juice is precisely adapted to the food we take in.

For the purpose of these experiments Pavlov investigated thousands of dogs, cats and mice, and he was always able to reproduce his findings. He demonstrated, for instance, that by merely seeing food, without actually eating or even tasting it, the whole of the intestinal tract begins to secretes its specific juice.

He made the following experiments: he cut through the oesophagus (food pipe) of a dog and stitched the upper end into the skin so that no food was able reach the stomach. Then he allowed the dog to eat, and the food came out of the hole in the oesophagus. He carried out another operation on this dog to obtain the excreted gastric juice. Although no food of any kind reached the stomach, the gastric juice and the intestinal juice were constituted exactly in accordance with the substance devoured by the dog. There must be something very wise at work here, which is not only able to judge the quality of the food, but also to synthesise the secreted juices according to the qualities of the food.

Pavlov speaks about nerves, reflexes and so on, but these are merely theories. What we can actually observe can be described in the following way: all the larger and smaller glands in our body – the pancreas, the gall bladder and the glands which line the wall of the intestines – collectively constitute a highly intelligent, discerning judge. Every kind of food we ingest is evaluated by these glandular chemists or alchemists with regard to its particular qualities.

The food is evaluated in minutest detail according to its quantity and quality. The secretions of all the intestinal glands are constituted according to this judgment. Now imagine what it means that, completely in darkness with respect to sensory awareness, we bear in us something you could call a judge – call it what you will, but we need to be aware that *something* is actively present – that this something is judging the food, and that according to this evaluation the appropriate gastric juices are instantly released.

Pavlov was able to show that our conscious sense organs too are connected with the intake of food. He carried out the following experiments: He trained dogs to eat only when a bell was rung, or when certain colours appeared in the room where they were kept. After the dogs had been trained, the mere ringing of the bell made the gastric juices flow, even without food being given. This shows that something that merely enters our sense organs, a sound, a certain colour, a certain smell, is able to stimulate the flow of the gastric juices. This knowledge is very important, not for developing new hypothesises, as Pavlov has done, but to enable us to take in these striking facts and to understand that our whole organism is so closely connected with our digestion. We cannot understand what nutrition means unless we take account of these facts.

On the one hand you have Pavlov's experiments. But there is another fact which very much stirred people's minds in the 1920s. This was not a scientific experiment, but a religious phenomenon that could be seen by anybody who wanted to witness it. This phenomenon was manifest in Therese of Konnersreuth.[1] She was a tailor's daughter in a small village in Bavaria, and had visions about the life and death of Christ. She was able to recall these visions and she even developed the stigmata.

After she had been having these visions for a certain time she stopped eating because she could no longer tolerate food – until she fasted completely. The only food she took was holy communion each Sunday. She did not grow weak as a result of this starvation; she was even able to do a certain amount of ordinary housework and some work on the land. She had normal faeces, and she passed water several times a day. Yet she took no food whatsoever and no water or other fluid. This was not a deception; a kind of religious experiment was conducted on this humble, simple human being. This special personality was able to live quite an ordinary life, but without eating food. What does this signify?

Both Pavlov's experiments and the religious experience of Therese of Konnersreuth indicate that there must be another source for keeping our body alive. Perhaps there is another way of understanding metabolism and digestion than the one usually taught by science.[2]

If we observe the gastric juices and the salivary juices, we can really begin to understand this precise judge, this intelligent sense, ruling all our glands within us. If we consider what Rudolf Steiner indicated in terms of the cosmic nutrition stream, an answer may begin to emerge which I shall now try to describe.

In the last two years of his life Rudolf Steiner unveiled more and more about this cosmic nutrition stream in a clear and convincing way. The fact is that our sense organs, our head, even our skin and our hair are not only what they appear to be. With the light of the sun, with the warmth, with all our sense perceptions, we not only receive the possibility of seeing, of hearing and of tasting the outer world; through all these sense organs we also receive a certain amount of life forces, etheric forces. The forces of warmth, light, sound and life stream into our body through the sense organs. In one of his lecture courses Rudolf Steiner gave a precise description of how these forces stream into us.[3] I do not want to go into details; I only want to give you a picture that you can contemplate.

Rudolf Steiner described how this cosmic nutrition stream constantly enters our sense organs, but not at the same rate at all times. From the sense organs – the eyes, ears, nose, mouth, etc. – it streams down into the body. It is through this cosmic nutrition stream that all our organs, our tissues and our cells are built up, because the etheric forces are the real and actual source, the true food of our body. If this is the case, why do we eat at all? If we have this cosmic nutrition and it feeds us, why do we depend so much on the amount and quality of the food we take in? The answer is that this cosmic nutrition stream is not flowing constantly at the same rate. I would like to give you a picture of its flowing. Imagine a smouldering fire in a fireplace, just smouldering, glowing, nothing more, and then imagine putting some wood on these glowing embers. The fire flares up and destroys the wood you threw in. A similar process takes place with the cosmic nutrition stream and the digestive process.

We know that a certain amount of warmth is always around our head. This raiment of warmth around our head is the smouldering fire that we carry within us. This smouldering fire starts to glow and to burn when we develop a fever, it starts to flame up. It also flames up the moment we start to eat, but then it burns differently to when we have a fever. It burns in such a way that through this flaming glow appearing around our head, the stream of cosmic nutrition pours itself into our sense organs in a much stronger flow.

From the sense organs the etheric forces of light, sound, warmth and life stream down on another level, but at the same time as the in-streaming food. The stream of earthly nutrition, which flows down, and the stream of cosmic nutrition, which enters through the head and the sense organs, these two streams flow downwards into our body. The cosmic stream becomes more and more material, and – imagine the different kinds of clouds Dr Lehrs spoke about – a certain kind of rain begins to precipitate out of the etheric clouds. This rain grows mightier and mightier and becomes none other than the flow of the gastric and intestinal juice. The cosmic nutrition stream can be measured by means of the quantity and the quality of the gastric and intestinal juices. This juice is ultimately the product of the streaming etheric forces. They stream in through every one of the gastric and intestinal glands, and it is these etheric forces that we earlier described as the 'judge'. This 'something' which is really assessing the quality and the quantity of the food we take in, this cosmic nutrition stream, is intelligent to the highest degree. These etheric forces respond directly without needing to contemplate or to be rational towards the food taken in. This radiating intelligence of etheric forces turns instantly into 'rain' within the intestinal tract.

This rain also falls on the outside of the walls of the intestinal tract. There is one vast sea or lake into which this rain streams, and this is the whole of the lymphatic system of our body. All the lymph vessels, with their lymphatic fluid, are essentially a collecting reservoir, into which the etheric forces of this rain of radiant etheric forces pours. Within the lymph vessels this rain turns into physical substance as intestinal juice within the boundaries of the intestinal walls. This cosmic nutrition stream passes through the whole of the organism down into the abdomen, and there it divides into the rain that pours down into the lymph stream, and into the rain that falls as intestinal juice in the intestinal tract.

If you observe how the convolutions of our intestines are surrounded by vast amounts of lymph vessels, you will appreciate why – in the absence of an awareness of the cosmic nutrition stream – it is believed nowadays that everything entering the intestinal tract goes through its walls and appears again inside the lymph vessels. If you imagine and consider the picture of the cosmic nutrition stream, these sun-rays that become rain inside our body, one part falling inside the intestine and the other part outside the intestinal wall, you can imagine how this cosmic nutrition stream actually acts and works.

In the previous lecture I said that faeces are the product of the intestinal juice. I have now shown that the whole of the gastric and intestinal juice is rain coming down from the cosmic nutrition stream. Ultimately, dung is the final product of the cosmic nutrition stream. The quality, power and etheric forces that are to be found in dung explain why dung is so absolutely necessary as a basis for agriculture. Dung is essentially the final product of the cosmic nutrition stream. It does not consist of physically and chemically modified foodstuffs, but is substance created out of the cosmic nutrition stream.

Cosmic forces and physical forces have mixed together to build up this intestinal milk. Is it now possible to discover a picture for everything I have attempted to describe? Nature has provided us with such a picture, showing us that there is not only physical nutrition, but also cosmic nutrition. Particularly as farmers, you are very connected with this picture in nature of the cosmic and the earthy nutrition stream. When you study ruminants, you find two closely connected families – the Bovidae (or bovids) and Cervidae (or deer family). If you look at two typical species of these families, the cow in the stable or meadow and the deer in the forests, cows have ordinary horns and deer have antlers. There is a big difference between these two families. These two types of anatomical structures are really polar opposites. Horns really derive from skin, whereas antlers derive from bone. The antlers are part of the skeleton; the horns are part of the skin.[4] Now observe and contemplate on these two species of animals.

The growth process of the horn is a very slow process. The skin is pushed up higher and higher, and so more and more of the horn appears. Hard, old substance is developed until the horn is formed, and this horn stays there for the whole of the animal's life. By contrast, the development of antlers is not a slow, gradual process that takes place in gradual steps, but is like a quick-fire process. Suddenly the bone breaks through the skull of a deer, piercing the skin, and grows for a short time. This antler is built up to last for only one year. The bone pierces the skin, and from the inside of the organism the skeleton turns outwards. While the horn is only an extension of the skin, a slow process, in the antlers the power and the fire of the blood causes this bone to grow. The antlers are surrounded by a large amount of blood, which builds them up. Imagine on the one hand wild deer running through the forest, their antlers sensing the atmosphere; and on the other hand the quietly grazing cow with its horns. Try to vividly imagine a cow – quietly eating and chewing; and then picture a deer, alert to every change around it, ready to run.

During the last twenty years certain investigations have been carried out on the embryonic development of roe-deer. After the egg is fertilised around October, the embryo grows for about ten days, and then stops growing. Then after about December 24 or 25, embryonic development gets going again. What does this signify? It shows that deer with their antlers are completely embedded in the etheric and spiritual forces of the surroundings. Even the embryo develops according to the spiritual festivals of the earth. Cows are the preservers of the physical nutrition stream. The horns hold together everything taking place within the cows' digestive tract. Deer run through the woods, wild and completely embedded in the spiritual and etheric atmosphere of the surroundings: deer bring down the cosmic nutrition stream with their antlers, showing the routes and pathways taken by the cosmic nutrition stream. If we could observe the cosmic nutrition stream descending, we would be able to see our whole head surrounded by a kind of antler structure. In these two families of animals, the bovids and the deer, Nature offers us a picture of the earthly and cosmic nutrition streams. If we are able to picture this in the right way we may learn to understand it.

What do we actually do when we take a stag's bladder and hang it up during the summer somewhere high up in a building?[25] You open the organ of such an animal, which is embedded in the cosmic nutrition stream; you make use of this vessel following its intrinsic nature by exposing it to the whole sunlit atmosphere. The horn, by contrast, is put into the earth, the dark ground of the soil. These are two opposite operations, and we may now be able to understand why this is done. We may learn to appreciate that the cosmic nutrition stream is a reality. With some effort we will not only come to understand it, but gradually to see and experience it to a greater or lesser degree.

There is something else I would like to mention. Last time several of you asked me to say something about alcohol and its forces. Does its nutritional value make any difference to the other food we eat? How do we take it in, and what does the organism do with alcohol? At the time I answered part of the question, but now, after speaking about the cosmic nutrition stream, I think I can say a little more.

I would like to remind you of intestinal milk, which comes about through the meeting of the cosmic and earthly nutritional streams: the cosmic intestinal rain and the food we have taken in. In this way a kind of milk is prepared. I call it a kind of milk because everything you can find in milk – proteins, fats, minerals – is also found in this intestinal milk. But consider alcohol; it is a very peculiar substance because it is the actual substance from which everything in our metabolism can be, and is prepared. Within the intestinal milk, tiny little droplets of alcohol appear and out of these drops anything can be built up. When living substance like fat, protein or carbohydrate is chemically broken down in so far that alcohol results from this destruction, everything can be built up from this alcohol again. Alcohol is for living matter what carbon is for living structure.

As we develop a better understanding of the nature of alcohol, we will also understand the focal point of the whole metabolism, because out of alcohol the body is able to make anything and everything.[6] Alcohol is turned into sugar, from sugar into fat, into every kind of organic ether, and in this way into any kind of protein.

We must learn to understand that there, beneath our diaphragm, there is only one substance – milk. This milk, about which I spoke in words and pictures once used by Rudolf Steiner when speaking about the Lemurian epoch, this worldwide milky atmosphere surrounding the earth, was the realm where the animals and the plants were really created. The same milky atmosphere, the same milk of creation, we have within us, and there are certain tiny spots of fire or lightning, which are nothing but alcohol. These drops of alcohol are the first centres, the focal points of these expanding substances, which develop into proteins, fats and carbohydrates. To understand this you have to see the whole human body and the metabolic processes as a great laboratory, not a laboratory as we have them today, but a laboratory corresponding to the whole of earth existence as it was in the Lemurian time. There is milk, and it is this milk that comes into existence through the flow of the cosmic nutrition stream. Out of this milk all the many thousands and thousands of different substances are prepared.

If, however, we follow the intake of carbon, nitrogen, oxygen, hydrogen and so on, we will not find anything that can enlighten our understanding of metabolism, because the way from intake to excretion is not a direct one. The excretions themselves can be investigated, but all that happens in between – that is so often not investigated in the laboratory – can be investigated if we take into account the creative forces descending and working in our body. Then we will understand that every intake of food amounts to a re-creation of the world.

Then we will understand that the 'Good Mummy', of which Paracelsus spoke, is not only found in milk, and that not only is urine the 'Bad Mummy', but that our cosmic nutrition stream is the 'Good Mummy', and that this 'Good Mummy' should be called the 'Wise Mummy' of the cosmic nutrition stream – this wise judge, who really always dispenses as much rain as is necessary for the soil of our digestion, as much rain and as many minerals as are necessary to destroy and to build up – to destroy what we take in, and to build up what is our whole organism.

In bodily existence, cosmically built up, there are two quiet spots – our brain, which gives us our consciousness, and the faeces, which – chiefly via the dung of our animals – gives consciousness to the soil.

Earthly and Cosmic Nutritional Streams in Human Beings and Plants

Four lectures for physicians and farmers at
Thornbury, Bristol, October 15 to 18, 1953

1 The Contrast Between the Senses and Digestion

Lecture 1, Thursday, October 15, 1953

It is particularly important that matters related to nutrition should become subject to discussion between doctors and farmers. I feel that during these mornings I should not be giving you a series of lectures, but that we should devote our time to studying together one of the most important problems concerning humankind, that of nutrition. I hope we will be able to consider this in connection with everything that Rudolf Steiner said on this subject in the course of his teaching. I think that nowadays we are insufficiently aware of the importance of this subject and of the deep layers of morality connected with it. The subject is at once mysterious and immense, and it can only be approached step by step.

I would like to say this by way of introduction. Those who have closely followed the writings of Rudolf Steiner's pupils during the last, say, ten years, will have noticed a great change, a change which, being a pupil of Rudolf Steiner myself, I have experienced within myself. To begin with, say, from 1925/26 until 1935, we were simply enthusiastic. We went out into the world proclaiming the threefold nature of man, the cosmic and earthly nutrition streams, how the theory of motor nerves is inapplicable, and so forth. We thought that we only needed to look around the corner, and these problems would easily be solved. We were too confident, and because of this overconfidence the problems were not tackled at a deep enough level. But now that we are in a position to survey all the material gathered together by anthroposophical writers and lecturers, and from Rudolf Steiner's published lectures, and also take into account what modern science has brought to light on a particular subject, we have become exceedingly cautious. We now consider every word Rudolf Steiner said much more carefully and with much deeper deliberation. As a result we gradually discovered how in fact all that Rudolf Steiner said in the course of the years on one or another subject fits together bit by bit until a more or less complete picture has been developed; only this picture is so tremendous that one is hardly able to comprehend it all at once.

If, for instance, we follow the subject of nutrition through Rudolf Steiner's lectures, we find that he started to speak about it as early as 1904 and 1905. There we find various remarks about a particular substance, milk. We also find that he indicates how complicated nutrition is. Then, during the succeeding years, he adds one piece of information after another to enhance our understanding; it is only during the last year of his teaching, in the lectures he gave to the farmers in Koberwitz, that he crowns it all when in the eighth lecture, he reveals that the whole of our organisation is not built up and nourished by the food we take in through our mouths but that this food, as nutritive substance, merely nourishes the brain; the organism as a whole, both in animal and in man, including claws, hands, muscles, bones and all our organs, is built up, and its invisible structure maintained by everything that comes to us as nourishment through our sense organs.[1] He elaborates on this point in one of the last lectures he gave, in September 1924, during the Pastoral Medical Course.[2]

We are left with this message, and it is now up to us to discover its real significance. What does it really mean if we say that the brain is essentially a dung-heap? This is what Rudolf Steiner said. In considering this lecture from the Agriculture Course –

and I think we will have to do this throughout our studies here – we should not simply accept this statement, but endeavour to understand it with our whole being. If, as intellectual beings, we can avoid feeling offended by such a statement, we will find that we can in fact easily understand that the brain is manure, excrement. Then there is another statement which Steiner made two years earlier in 1923: 'The human brain is really nothing but hardened milk juice.'[3]

Now let us compare these two statements. On the one hand Rudolf Steiner said: 'The brain is nothing but hardened milk juice,' and elsewhere he said it is the end product of a process which started in our intestines; that it is completed, hardened manure. Only if you go through many of Rudolf Steiner's lectures and find your way through all the statements and descriptions he gave about milk, can you gradually begin to see why dung and milk should be more or less closely related. I am saying all this as a kind of introduction to our work; let us now take the eighth lecture of the Agriculture Course as our background material.

Now we shall start with something familiar. We know that the process of photosynthesis takes place in the green leaf of a plant in such a way that light streams in from above and carbon dioxide enters from below.

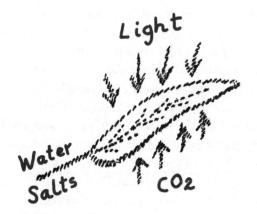

The cells of the upper part of the leaf are arranged in parallel in such a way that the light can stream in easily through the transparent surface. Underneath, sponge-like cells take up (I do not say suck up) carbon dioxide. The third process is the influx of water and salts taken up by the roots. Thus there are three processes: light from above, carbon dioxide from below, and water and salt flowing in through the roots, so that the process of photosynthesis, the formation of special plant substances (mostly carbohydrates), can take place.

This process is, in its finer details, still a complete mystery to modern science. We do not know how this process comes about because light is quite simply not understood in the right way: it is seen merely as a source of energy and nothing else. In his *Metamorphosis of Plants,* Goethe said of the leaf, 'The whole plant is nothing but leaf.' The roots are leaf, the flowers are leaf. The plant, as an archetypal being, consists of nothing but leaf and the metamorphosis of leaves. If this applies to forms, should it not also apply to processes? Thus we may ask, how does this process of photosynthesis, or assimilation, metamorphose in the various parts of the plant?

If we take the whole plant, the roots are below, the leaves in the middle and the flowers above. Is there any way of understanding how light and carbon dioxide metamorphose in the upper and in the lower part of the plant? When we look at a plant and follow this process of metamorphosis, going from the green leaf up into the coloured petal, we see that the coloured petal no longer has the power of photosynthesis; nor does the root. Only the leaf has it. To call the leaf the food-factory of the plant is of course utterly wrong, because it gives a totally different meaning to the phenomenon. The leaves do something that is lost to the roots on the one hand, and to the flowers on the other. But why? If we try to transform the green leaf into the coloured petal in our imagination, as an inner soul metamorphosis, we will experience that the flower can no longer freely accept the light. The leaf is given up to the light, and therefore light enters unhindered. But the flower, as it were, hinders the light and reflects it. Only because light does not penetrate but is reflected, refused entry, because the flower does not want the light, does the flower appear in its coloured beauty. I do not wish to add any psychological comments here, but you may be able to understand that beauty always entails developing a certain element of rejection. This is what the flower does.

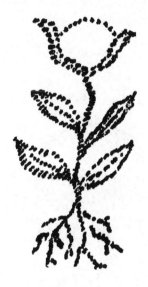

The root, on the other hand, has something else. Usually the root, if it is in its proper realm, is not colourless, but is dark – brown or black. It is not rejection that is associated with this colour, but rather a kind of sucking, receiving, a kind of taking in. This arises from the carbohydrate process, where it descends into the sphere of the root. And now you can see how the leaf processes of the plant change upwards into the flower process which rejects, and downwards into the root process which absorbs and sucks in. If this is properly understood, we can go one step further: imagine changing the leaf from a flat structure into a kind of sphere.

The upper side is the realm where the light out of space streams in; the underside is the dark side where carbon dioxide nourishes the leaf. It would be quite wrong to say that nutritional, digestive or metabolic processes of any kind go on in a plant. Such processes lie entirely outside the plant kingdom, because the plant merely provides a kind of scaffold for the meeting of cosmic powers and cosmic substances. The plant is in its essence the meeting place of cosmic and earthly forces.

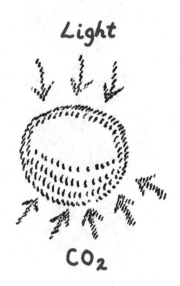

If this archetypal image of the plant process alters in such a way that animal or man starts to develop, the underside becomes invaginated like a ball which has been pressed in, and we see the formation which is commonly called the gastrula.

The round sphere of the leaf has now progressed to the archetypal form of a simple animal. On the upper side sensory processes arise, and in the lower, invaginated part, digestion and nutrition processes begin. In this way we have made the step from the plant to the animal. This step has arisen from a differentiation between nutrition and digestion, which are processes that take in the substances of the outer world, and sensory processes, which reject the world. The lower part accepts, the upper part rejects.

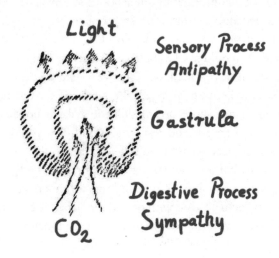

Once we understand this, we can begin to understand what Rudolf Steiner referred to in the first chapters of the book *(Extending Practical Medicine)* which he and Dr Ita Wegman wrote at about the time of the Koberwitz Course; here for the first time he wrote about different conditions of substances: physical substance, living substance and sensitive substance. He wrote about sensitive substance in the following way: nutrition and digestion are only possible when the substance, the sensitive substance, develops sympathy with the surrounding world; and sensory processes are only possible when sensitive substance develops antipathy towards the surrounding world. We must learn to become conscious, with all our thinking, feeling and will, of the fact that sensory processes are connected with rejection and antipathy, and that nutrition and digestion processes are connected with sympathy.

Normally when describing how the world comes towards us via our sensory processes, and how we go out into the world with our limbs, we have a half-conscious, dreamy idea that we are sympathetic to the outside world in our upper organism and antipathetic in our lower organism. This idea is deeply rooted in every one of us: throughout our school and university education it is instilled into us that our sense organs are passive, and do nothing but rest and allow the world to enter in. This is what physiologists would have us believe. The truth is just the reverse. We see, we hear, we smell, we taste, we touch, we experience the world simply because we reject the world. If we did not reject the world, if our sense organs did not make it possible for us continually to go out and resist the world, we would never be able to see, to hear, to listen, to taste, to smell, and still to remain ourselves. By contrast, whenever food enters the body, a process of sympathy is involved. We must learn to understand this, not simply intellectually, but with our whole being. We would never 'get in touch' with the food we eat, if all the sensitive substance in our body did not take this food and make it its own.

Do not think that sympathy simply means embracing something, being kind, nice and good. If for instance, I should find it necessary to be sympathetic towards somebody, and hit him in the face, it might be one of the strongest means of demonstrating my sympathy. For the fact is that every contact with the world is an act of sympathy. There, something happens: karma is enacted. This can come about by embracing someone, but also by striking someone.

Antipathy does not bring about anything real when a meeting takes place. This is the second point that we shall now have to consider. In the sensory process, it is antipathy that continually changes the world, which it rejects by turning it into an image. Our sense organs do not give us the world itself, but only an image of the world. We have an image of the world – which is of course a true, not a false image, as modern physiology and psychology would have us believe – but it is nevertheless an image. There is a very simple experiment you can do. It is not very pleasant but it is revealing. If you spin around more and more quickly, you will suddenly notice that all you see of the world is an image, because it moves in an entirely different way from you yourself; and then when you stop, you will find that the table, the walls and the ceiling go on moving round you, for they are nothing but images.

On the other hand, in order to help you understand what I mean by rejection, consider the following: in the course of the evolution of humankind we have acquired the capacity to walk upright, to adopt a position whereby we contravene the laws of gravity. We are able to overcome gravity thanks to a very complicated process culminating in the formation of our organ of balance, in our three semi-circular canals.[4] What have we gained by acquiring this equilibrium? We have in fact emancipated ourselves from the forces which make our earthly globe turn on its own axis and revolve around the sun, and make the whole planetary system move through space. The plants are given up to these forces, and therefore their growth patterns reveal the movements of the earth, the planets and the sun. These movements have built the plants. We, on the other hand, have emancipated ourselves from these forces and therefore we always know through our own experience, that up is where our head is, and down is where our feet are. Neither the rotation of the earth nor the movement of the earth round the sun nor the movement of the whole planetary system through cosmic space is within us any longer: we have rejected them, and we know where up is. In the same way we have rejected the light, and therefore the colours and the forms of the world appear to us. We have rejected sound, and therefore we can hear. We reject substance, and this rejection makes it possible for us to smell and taste.

Perhaps we can now understand why Rudolf Steiner, when speaking about the head, always calls it the *antipathetic system*.[5] This system, which is closed off as it were, which has formed itself and made itself independent, this head is essentially an embodiment of antipathy, which has withdrawn from the whole of the surrounding world. Because the head is removed from the world around us, the world appears to us, and our head becomes a kind of mirror for this world. With our nutritive system, with our digestive tract, with everything we need in order to take in nourishment, we accept the world, we receive it sympathetically. We only want to unite with the world, and in so doing, overcome it. But this is, of course, the first stage. It is a stage that applies to the invertebrate animals.

If we go one step further, into the world of the vertebrates – animals with a backbone, a heart and a closed circulatory system – and especially if we enter the human kingdom, this does not cease to be true. However, to understand the fundamental human sensory processes on the one hand, and the digestive and nutritive processes on the other, something else needs to be added. If we recollect how we considered the plant, the flower and the root, and how we tried to understand the flower as being on the way to containing digestive processes, we will suddenly find ourselves confronted with the question, did not Rudolf Steiner say just the opposite? And I have to say: yes, he did!

Now we have to ask ourselves the following question: in the plant we have the flowery-sensory pole and the root-nutritive pole; on the other hand, Rudolf Steiner said that the roots are connected with our head organisation, and the flowers with our metabolic-nutritive-digestive organisation. Why?

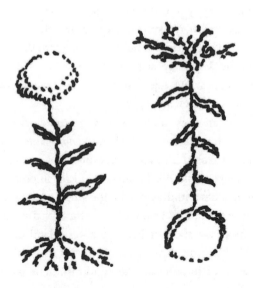

Let us consider the human eye. The human eye has an outer covering – I am describing it now from a particular point of view – the sclera, which at the front of the eye, develops into the cornea that becomes transparent so that light can enter. Within this eyeball, formed by the sclera, there is the choroid layer and, within that, as an inner layer, the retina. Because it consists of nerve tissue, the retina has until now been considered to be the organ responsible for the process of seeing. The familiar idea, still found in every textbook, is that a candle held in front of the eye produces an image of the candle on the retina.

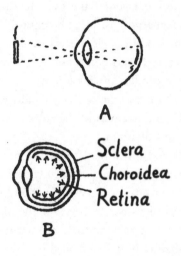

This is certainly possible. And there is no doubt that if you examine an animal's eye, you will find that the last shapes the eye saw are imprinted on the retina. But if you investigate this retina in both humans and animals more closely, you will find that the retina consists of about one hundred million tiny little organs, nerve organs, which, owing to their different shapes, are described as rods and cones. You can imagine how tiny they are if you consider that there are about a hundred million of them in each eye. But one thing, dear friends, is most astounding:

quite understandably, these rods and cones have been credited with the process of seeing because it was thought that they are tiny little mirrors; this is probably true. They function more or less as some kind – and I emphasize kind – of mirror. But the remarkable thing is that these mirrors should not face outwards towards the world, but away from it. It is as if I were to look at you with my back turned.

If one tries to discuss this with scientists, they will say that it is very difficult, because there is simply no accounting for this structure; they can only shrug their shoulders and say, well, the rods and cones must know what they are doing! In fact, they face into the choroid layer of the eyeball. And why? Because there they have something to see. The choroid layer is the layer that carries all the blood vessels – arteries and veins – that stream into the eye. The rods and cones are in fact mirrors in exactly the same way the papillae of our tongue are mirrors. They eat substances in a most complicated way. And the function of the choroid layer is to receive part of the cosmic nutrition stream. I will say more about this later.

In vertebrates and in humans, sensory processes are accompanied by digestive processes, and only when both are seen together can we learn to approach the real problem. We find the same thing in the digestive process; for the digestive processes in humans and the higher animals are permeated by sensory processes. We shall only understand this if we realise that both above and below, we find nutritional and sensory processes. Of course, at one pole the sensory process is in the foreground of consciousness.

Discussion

Question: You described how the senses reject the world. Otherwise there would be no perception of the world, no beholding. The world would simply stream into us. And that is an antipathetic movement one makes. I found it difficult to understand how, when you give your friend a blow in the face that could be considered a sympathetic act. Unless all one's outer movements, such as walking on the ground, are also sympathetic acts. Could you say a little more about that?

Karl König: In his lectures on psychology in 1910, and also in his lectures on Anthroposophy in 1909, Rudolf Steiner described the fundamental activity of the human soul thus: the human soul has two tendencies: antipathy and sympathy.[6] On this point, he went into great detail. When, a few years later, he revealed the threefold human being, one was able to understand sympathy and antipathy as the two fundamental functions of our rhythmical organisation.[7] It is our rhythmical system that carries all our feelings. In our feelings we develop sympathetic and antipathetic emotions. If antipathy goes to the extreme, the upper system predominates; if sympathy becomes too strong, the lower system predominates.

Then Rudolf Steiner went one step further in 1919, when addressing the teachers of the Waldorf School for the first time, he gave his basic course *Study of Man* or *Foundations of Human Experience*. In the very first lectures he gave the following picture: when we approach the earth [on our way to incarnation], we bring with us all the antipathy forces by which we have freed ourselves from the cosmic world. As he once expressed it, antipathy is then so strong that the cosmos spits out our head; we are born.

With these antipathy forces — through prolonged pondering and meditation it is possible to understand this — we turn our sense impressions of the world around us into images. This means that it no longer has reality in itself. If you imagine what it would be like if we only saw, heard, smelled and tasted the world, that the world was for us nothing but perception — then we would have no will to exist, no will to live. We would simply be nothing but a sphere of mirrors; things would move around us, appear to us as a result of antipathy, with our head as a mirror. But we would have no impulse whatsoever to act, to live, to exist. You find such a condition nowadays among children and adults as a neurotic condition. This can even go one step further: some people today, instead of experiencing the world, only experience books; they retire from the world into the imaginary garden of the printed word.[8] All this is a manifestation of the antipathy we bring with us from our life between death and rebirth.

But you see that we always have to make holes in the image of the world provided by our senses. And we can do this only with the power of sympathy. This power continually brings about the destruction of the world of the senses. Instead of creating images, this power is the origin of what Rudolf Steiner in these lectures called the germ. With this germ within the seed we enter our life after death, carrying with us the new destiny that we have built up. The sympathy forces are not only the loving ones. The loving forces are one aspect of sympathy, but sympathy is actually everything that connects itself with the world, takes hold of the world, builds the world as well as destroys it. You can't build anything without first destroying something. If you embark on some new work, you first have to put aside all that has been done before. You may incorporate a few seeds of tradition, but first you have to create chaos. Have you never experienced how an angry word spoken to another human being may suddenly clear the air? It may initially darken the air, and then a few more cross words are needed. Expressing sympathy means getting in touch as closely as possible with the world, and creating seeds, germs, for the future. This is how I understand the sympathy forces.

What does it matter if sympathy is expressed, for instance, as a blow, if it is appropriate in the situation? It will in any case find its compensation after death, in kama loka! And in this way I may be creating the seeds of a potential future friendship. Please don't think that I am advocating going through the world like that. Not at all! But you can't plant without breaking the ground. Ploughing is as much an act of sympathy as sowing, the one being more gentle, the other more energetic. There is no alternative unless you were to become a Buddhist, in which case you withdraw as far as possible into the forces of antipathy. We must grasp what Rudolf Steiner meant when he describes the forces of sympathy in this way.

Since the beginning of the nineteenth century, when the great physiologist Johannes Müller announced his theory of sense perception, in which he maintained that every sense organ can receive stimuli only from the outer world, transforming these into perceptions, the scientific conception of the human being has become completely misguided.[9] When this law became accepted, the inescapable conclusion was that everything we experience through our senses is merely personal imagination. Colours don't actually exist, neither does sound nor smell nor taste. All these are simply created by our sense organs, while the reality around us is an empty, colourless and soundless space, where certain vibrations simply stimulate our sense organs. From these stimuli we create the imaginary world in which we live. This is still considered to be true, although we do not accept it in practice. Theoretically it is accepted by science, but scientists themselves do not accept it in practice, because they treat their sense experiences as if they were real. I consider Johannes Müller to have been a great man, and it was only the fact that he lived in the nineteenth century which induced him to formulate this law in such a way that it had these disastrous consequences. But there is something else behind this, which I believe we must gradually learn to see. And now I would like to elaborate on some of the points I have already touched on in my lecture.

When we eat, we take in carbohydrates, fats, proteins, salt

and a great variety of other substances. These we ingest in the form of many different plants, animals and minerals. We put a great variety of substances into our mouths. Yet when we start digesting, we reduce the variety to a unity, we produce what is called chyme in the small intestine. Chyme is no longer the sum total of the different kinds of food which entered our body when we ate; it is a generalised, unified fluid, into which the different kinds of substances have dissolved. Chyme is a universalised (homogenised) substance; salt and plants and meat have relinquished their individual character, transforming into a homogenous substance. Therefore we can compare chyme with milk and assert that both are universal substances in which their constituents have laid aside some or all of their individuality and become bound together interdependently.

At the opposite pole we have the sensory processes. And now I must say something that may initially surprise many of you. For many years I asked myself what made Johannes Müller formulate this law in the way he did. It is at odds with everything he accomplished, for he was in fact clairvoyant; in describing his own soul processes, he described clairvoyant experiences.

Earlier I described the transformation of the leaf into the gastrula: how at one pole light is rejected, and through this rejection the first basic sensory experience arises; and how at the other pole carbon dioxide is sucked in and becomes the fundamental process of nutrition. This stage of evolution has its roots far back in the past, during the Old Saturn stage of evolution, where the first beginnings of the sense organs were created. There the sense process began. Our colour vision is due to our having developed eyes; our hearing of sounds is due to our having developed ears; our capacity to smell various scents is due to our having developed noses. Not only the individual organs, but also the smelling process, the seeing process, the hearing process must be taken into account. The more the processes of seeing, hearing, smelling and tasting unfolded, the more the outer world became separated out as sense perception and thereby individualised. What lies behind our sensory organs is what creates the differentiation we now see in the world around us.

This differentiation between sensory organs and the world as perceived by them has evolved until it has reached its present state. Now it is no longer a question of individualisation, but of maintaining the differentiation that has been achieved. Only as long as we keep this differentiating, antipathetic process going, does the world continue to exist for us in its diversity. This process is what we call sense perception.

Now to move on to something else, which I referred to in my lecture this morning from a different point of view. Rudolf Steiner described our head organisation and our lower organisation in the following way: he said that our head organisation is actually a synthetic organisation, it is synthesised, whereas our lower organisation is analysed. What is pressed together in our head is differentiated in our lower organisation. This is the first and fundamental statement in his Curative Education course *(Education for Special Needs)*.

In our abdomen we carry our liver and our spleen, our gall bladder, our small intestines, our kidneys and all our different organs. But in the head, there is a single organ, the brain. If you investigate the brain, you will find that it has qualities of liver, of intestines, of spleen, of kidney. All these qualities, which in the abdomen work through their separate organs, are synthesised in the brain into one organ.

This is now apparently the exact opposite of what I told you before. Because our head organisation is in itself a synthesis, it can maintain the differentiation of the sense perceptions. And because our abdominal organisation is itself differentiated, it is continually able to create the synthesis of chyme. I said that chyme is essentially to be considered as milk. To take the image a step further, we can now understand that the brain, in the synthetic head organisation, is solidified milk. So you see that what is a *process* below becomes *form* above, and what is *form* below becomes *process* above. The organs of our metabolic system are the differentiation of the synthesising of the differentiating forces in our sense perceptions. Now I can point again to the diagram of root and flower. We shall go into this in greater detail later.

Thomas Weihs: It is remarkable that the picture of digestion, which Dr König has built up, is also a picture of the modern scientific way of thinking. In describing the variety of colours scientifically, this variety has been reduced to quantitative difference within a single quality. And so it is in all the sciences. Science sets out with the aim of finding a single law, which manifold phenomena obey. This is actually digestion. And I think this can help us to understand why, at a time when science has made such tremendous progress, one phenomenon has increased appallingly, and that is fear. If we think of our grandparents, it is quite obvious that the main difference between them and an average person of today is that they felt secure and were comparatively free of fear. That this increase in fear should occur now is very striking. Science is not a process belonging to our head organisation, but is in fact digestion, and it follows that quite clinically the picture of fear, or the organic equivalent of fear, should suddenly appear.

Goethe did not attempt to discover which species of animals could be grouped together in one class, or which different phenomena obeyed one law; he tried to discover what distinguishes one phenomenon from another, and how it can be metamorphosed into the next. That is true nerve-sense activity, maintaining the differentiation of the diversity or manifoldness. The scientific method does not lead to knowledge in the sense of experienced insight, but to control. It does not require a great deal of insight into one's own body to know that eating, particularly digesting, is the one process by which we assert our power over the world. When I have eaten a bit of cabbage, I have destroyed it, and I am, as it were, the victor. That is what happens to our experience of the natural world when subjected to the reductionist methodology of orthodox science.

Karl König: This is a most important point. Because time and again you will see that in considering nutrition, it is no longer a scientific question, it is a question of morality. Nutrition has the deepest moral implications. Therefore it is so important that farmers in particular should learn to view it in the right way. During the first years after Rudolf Steiner spoke of this subject, we went out into the world proclaiming our knowledge about the cosmic and the earthly nutrition streams. And people asked, quite justifiably: but if we are cosmically nourished, why produce proper vegetables, if we do not use them anyhow? They will only feed a tiny part of the brain, so why worry? And this was a perfectly justified question, which we did not put to ourselves because we were not sufficiently honest with ourselves – not because we were dishonest people, but because we were over-enthusiastic, and therefore failed to look into it properly. And only gradually are we now learning to understand the moral side of this problem. Without re-establishing morality in cultivating proper food, no true moral rearmament will be possible. When we eat cabbage, flour or whatever, grown with chemical fertiliser, we simply take in immoral forces, which we then have to struggle to overcome.[10]

2 Nutrition in Digestion and the Senses

Lecture 2, Friday, October 16, 1953

Our task yesterday was not an easy one, either for you or for me. I think it will be still more complicated today. On such occasions, Rudolf Steiner would often tell the story of the Spanish king who was very cross because the world was arranged in such a complicated way, saying, 'If I were God, I would have made things much simpler.' But as we are not God, we must accept the situation as it is – and it is a very complicated one indeed. It is so complicated in fact that I must warn you not to expect that, by the end of this conference, you will know exactly what the cosmic and the earthly nutrition streams are. At present, it is not even possible for us to know exactly how, for instance, the process of seeing or the act of hearing works. Rudolf Steiner once said that it has taken a hundred years to develop a physiology of the senses, and it is not even correct yet.[1] We have to accept this. Whatever we are able to do at the moment is only a contribution, which can help us to take one further step; without such attempts, we cannot build the pathway that ultimately will make it possible to reach the goal.

This is one reason why you will find apparent contradictions in many of Rudolf Steiner's discussions on various subjects; these are necessary contradictions. For instance, in two different lectures on nutrition which he gave to the workmen at

181

the Goetheanum – one on January 23, 1924, and the other on October 20, 1923[2] – which probably are familiar to many of you, he speaks about protein, carbohydrates, fat, etc. In fact in each one of these two lectures he says entirely different things about these substances. In the second half of this morning, we will be able to discuss this. Here we have a typical kind of contradiction, which we are able to resolve by our own attempts at understanding. We will be able to see how such apparent contradictions can simply dissolve into a better understanding on a higher level. Therefore, I would ask you to please take all I say today as an attempt, and not as a solution. I am very conscious that it is merely a small contribution to this vast question – the cosmic and earthly nutrition streams. Nevertheless, I think that farmers should contemplate this tremendous riddle at least once, possibly every time they come together.

What I tried to make a little more comprehensible yesterday was the fact that in our sensory system we also harbour digestive processes, and in our digestive tract we harbour sensory processes. Both processes work in an intimate interrelationship. Above, sense perception is intimately connected with digestion; and below, digestion is intimately connected with sense perception. In the second half of the morning, I tried to show how the sensory world is differentiated, but has as its organ the head system, which in itself is synthetic; and how below, the digestive organs are differentiated, while the chyme, which is formed from the different food substances, is something which we could call a universalised substance. It is, as it were, to be considered as a kind of milk. And what we carry within our head, our brain, is, according to Rudolf Steiner's description, consolidated milk. If we now imagine these two aspects together, the chyme from below and the brain from above, we will immediately understand that it is just in the sphere of the rhythmic system that humans and animals produce the ordinary, common milk. This is just an introductory picture.

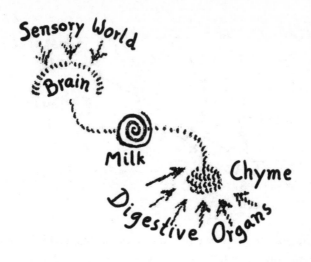

Now we can go one step further. We can ask: where is the actual cleft where sensory and digestive processes split from one another? Where is it that our whole organisation is divided into two parts, an upper and a lower one? This occurs at a quite specific place, located between our eyes and our mouth. Diagrammatically this could be represented as follows: we find that four sense organs are distributed in perfect harmony within the face; our eyes and ears, our nose and mouth make our face what it is. If we study the form of these sense organs, we will see that two of them have their main axis in the horizontal plane, and two of them have their main axis in the vertical plane. As soon as we start to contemplate this, we find that it conceals something special. Above are the eyes, and below, the mouth, with tongue, teeth and all that belongs to it. If we follow the eye anatomically, via the optic nerve into the brain, and the mouth into the whole digestive system, we will see that there is a correspondence between these two structures.

If we then remember Rudolf Steiner's diagram of the twelve sensory processes, we may also remember that seeing corresponds to Capricorn, and tasting stands under Sagittarius.[3]

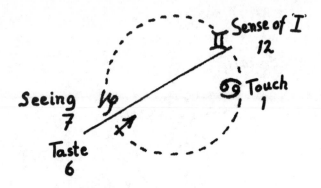

Opposite to these we find the sense of touch and the sense of I-in-the-other, or sense of the other as embodied subject. If we consider all the twelve sensory channels, we can now see how the line dividing the sense of sight from the sense of taste, when continued, becomes the line dividing the sense of touch (1) from the highest of our senses, the sense of I as other (12). And we become aware how there is something in this division between taste and sight, which involves all our sensory processes. For one might say, this line was drawn, and 'their eyes were opened.' At that moment, Adam began to look into the world above the line – and the whole *maya* of sensory existence came into being. Below this line, nutrition started in the way we have had to carry it on ever since.

This split has bundled together all our lower senses, but has also made it possible for all our higher senses to unfold. Perhaps this is an indication as to why it was said that when the Tree of Knowledge was given to Adam and Eve, the Tree of Life was taken away. The Tree of Knowledge opened at the moment when, to put it pictorially, the eye was separated from the mouth.

Studying the human anatomy of the eye and the mouth, shows not a striking difference, but rather a striking similarity between these two organs.

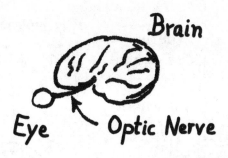

I will not go into details but I must indicate some things that will be valuable for your further study. When you consider the whole digestive tract, you will find it is built up in a most wonderful way. In it the same two forces are working which also build the plant. The digestive tract is built up so that in certain places everything is contracted, shortened, and nodes are formed; at other places it is expanded and elongated. Let us start with the mouth, which is a round, hollow organ. From the mouth, the oesophagus (food pipe) descends. There you can see the first shortening and elongation. Then comes the stomach, the second shortening or contraction, and then a tremendous elongation in the small intestine. Then, finally, there is the large intestine, where shortening and elongation have in a way grown together. Thus there are three steps: First step, mouth and oesophagus; second step, stomach and small intestine; third step, the extended, hollow formation of the large intestine. Thus there is a rhythm of short-long, short-long, which underlies the rhythmic structure of our digestive tract.

The mouth represents this whole structure as a seed, as it were. Consider the tongue within the mouth and, on the tongue, the different papillae, the sensory organs of taste. Any upset in the stomach or small intestines will show itself on the surface of the tongue; the tongue is a concentration of what exists, in expanded form, throughout the whole length of the intestine. For this reason, great physicians like Wilhelm Heinrich Schüssler,

185

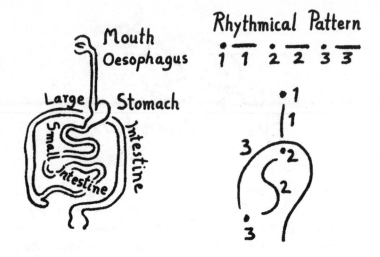

Samuel Hahnemann and others have administered remedies simply by placing them on certain parts of the tongue.[4] There is also a particular disease of the human blood, connected with the stomach, where only the tip of the tongue is affected.[5] Once we know more about general anatomy and particularly about the finer anatomy of the tongue, we will be able to draw the whole geography of the intestinal tract upon it.

In the mouth the rows of teeth – both the upper and lower – form a kind of arc. And the same arc can again be found in the large intestine. We can see how the tongue within the arc of the teeth is repeated in the small intestine, duodenum, etc., which are surrounded by the large intestine. Even in the finer anatomy of the large intestine we can find more or less the same number of structural units as we find in the sixteen upper and lower teeth.

There is another thing that can give some idea of how many things are involved. Where the small intestine joins the large intestine, the appendix is located. The appendix is a kind of lymph gland; it is, essentially, a tonsil. Where the arc of the teeth is connected with the beginning of the pharynx, we find the ton-

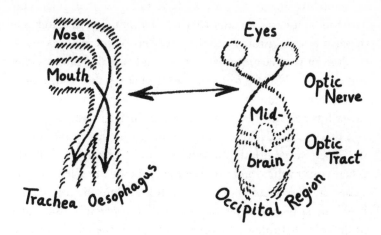

sils. This means that exactly the same structure is found above and below. We should therefore not be surprised that tonsillitis is frequently accompanied by appendicitis, which is like a tonsillitis down below, or vice-versa.

Now that we have grasped this, we can move on to a further anatomical study and consider the organisation of the eye. Our two eyes are connected to the optic nerve.

Without going into too much detail, the optic nerves join together underneath the brain, and then split up again, as it were. They split up inside the brain and then have a very long journey, running right through the brain to the other side of the head, terminating in the occipital region of the brain. Along the way, they send connecting fibres especially to the thalamic region, the mid-brain. Applying the idea of metamorphosis, we find here a repetition of the whole digestive system, only that this is a hardened form of what is soft and mobile below; it is a synthesised form of what is analysed below.

There are, as it were, two mouths, which are our two eyes. The one has split into two, or the two have merged into one. It is not difficult to understand that our eyelids and our lips are somehow the same, only we have to realise that in fact our lower lids are the metamorphosis of our upper lip and our upper lids are equivalent to the lower lip. You can also see the wisdom in language, in that 'lip' and 'lid' are almost the same. But try to see it in the following way: what is below is mirrored in the organisation above, and vice-versa. So that really the lower lids are the organic, living mirror image of our upper lip, and the upper lids are the organic mirror image of our lower lip. Open your mouth, and you see the white rows of teeth. Open your eyelids, and you see the white of the sclera. In the same way, the opening of our mouth leads into the throat, and in the most beautifully refined and subtle structure, the pupil of the eye, surrounded by the diaphragm of the iris, leads into the interior of the eye.

In the eyes of many of the vertebrates, especially birds, and also the embryological development of the eyes of higher animals as well as of humans, we find a structure called the fan extends into the eyeball. It is a kind of conglomeration of blood vessels, which project into the eyeball. As it is filled with blood, scientists have decided that this fan is a kind of central heating radiator for the eye which keeps it warm; otherwise the poor eye would be far too cold. In humans, this system of blood vessels has gradually disappeared, making it possible for the retina to become a flat lining on the inner eyeball. This fan is in fact a metamorphosis of the tongue. It sticks out into the eye in exactly the same way the tongue sticks into the mouth. The human eye is formed in such a way that the 'tongue' has disappeared. The eyes are really like two mouths and two pharynxes.

If we move from the mouth downwards to the oesophagus, we find another structure. Above we have the nose, and below, the nasal passage crosses over the pharynx to go into the larynx and the trachea. This again is an organic metamorphosis of what is above. Up to the crossing of the optic nerves there is the structure that corresponds to the pharynx. Up to the mid-brain runs a metamorphosis of the oesophagus, and the mid-brain itself corresponds to the stomach. The parietal and occipital region can be compared to the small and large intestines.

Recent physiological studies have shown that wherever there are nerve endings, minute quantities of a very complex substance, acetylcholine, are discharged. This means that even up there, where the optic nerve terminates, a kind of very subtle and fine secretion takes place of minute quantity, but in itself similar to what I have previously described as digestive function. The eyes, with the optic nerves and their continuation into the brain, are in fact essentially a metamorphosis of the digestive tract: only the one runs from the mouth downwards, while the other runs from the eyes backwards.

All this is really just a kind of elaboration of what I said yesterday. And I hope that it is becoming ever more clear that, both above and below, sensory processes and digestion are found together; only the relationship between these two processes is different above and below. When we start to eat various kinds of food, this act of eating lies with respect to our consciousness more or less entirely within the sensory sphere. Within our mouth we have a number of different sense perceptions, not only the sense of taste, but connected with it the sense of smell. We know how sometimes, when we really eat – rather than gulp – our food, smelling and tasting are intermingled. But we also sense warmth and cold; we have the sense of touch and connected with it the sense of movement, because when we eat we know exactly where our tongue is, how our jaws are placed, how we are biting, chewing and swallowing.

So all these sense perceptions, the sense of touch, the sense of life – whether we like something or don't like it – the sense of movement, the sense of smell, the sense of taste and the sense of warmth are all involved simultaneously when food is taken in. Then, gradually, this perception disappears. We can still follow our food into the gut, and sometimes the sense of touch and the sense of warmth may persist into our intestines, but gradually our sense perception dies down. Only if we are ill do we have a kind of sensation in our organs, but this is not normal. The act of digestion completely disappears from the world of sense impressions.

On the other hand, in the upper realm, the act of digestion is unconscious from the start. We have no awareness of it. Sense perception has become so important, especially through our eye's power of vision, that it takes a tremendous amount of reorientation to imagine that our nervous system, insofar as it is connected with our senses, is not really actively engaged in the act of sense perception; that it is in fact engaged in the act of digestion. Our retina, our optic nerve and the optic nervous tract together form one of the nerve systems by which the world that we take in through our senses as an act of nutrition is taken up and digested. If we took away the eyes, our sense perception would have nowhere to settle down on, as it were. You may be able to understand how our sense organs are really just the thrones on which sense perception sits. When I look out into the world, when I listen to the world, what am I actually doing? With my higher organisation, my 'I' and my astral body, I am outside, and this world which I see is mine, because I am in it. But all this activity must be rooted somewhere, must have a seat, a throne. And in continually encountering this throne, in sitting on this throne with my higher organisation, I become aware: I see, I hear, I smell, I taste.

From the perspective of earth reality, it is much easier to understand this whole process, because things have to come to meet me; to understand that the tongue is just as much a throne as the eye is much easier because I realise that I – as a higher entity – and matter have to meet, and then I am taste, and then I am smell. I and the world outside of me, we sit together as the 'image without reality' on the throne of the eye. But the eye itself, while providing this seat, is at the same time an organ of digestion. For not only do I see this world around me, but within this world (although it is nothing but an image) there live etheric forces, there live entities which come to me from the cosmos, from all those spheres which are filled with light. It is this, then, which is digested, accepted by the retina, accepted by the organ of hearing, accepted by the tongue.

Now we can see where the doors and entrance gates of the cosmic nutrition stream are: everywhere where the neuroepitheliums (the sensory cells) of our sense organs are distributed. These are the entrance gates for the cosmic nutrition stream, and these gates are actually the 'seats' to which the sense perceptions for our astral body and 'I' can attach themselves. The same holds good for the lower part of our organism. Here too we start with sense perception, and then descend into unconsciousness, lose the diversity of sense impressions, and combine all matter and substance by breaking it down into chyme.

Discussion

Karl König: Now I would like to consider the process of eating. When we take in food, the different substances that make it up, and the different sense perceptions by which we are aware of it, are both gradually dissolved by the various intestinal juices within the stomach and the small intestine, turning into chyme. I already tried to explain how chyme is in fact a kind of milk. But what kind of milk is it? What difference is there between this intestinal chyme and real milk? Rudolf Steiner said – and this conforms to what science has discovered – that all outer substance that we take in has to lose its individuality. We cannot take in cabbage, we cannot take in pork, we cannot take in spinach, potatoes and all the rest, for if we did, we would not be able to keep our own individuality intact. Therefore we break them down and destroy them. We wipe out their individualised existence and mould and change them into chyme. Chyme is a substance that I consider to be entirely physical or mineralised. Both the etheric and the astral forces, both the sensitive substance of the animal kingdom and the living substance of the plant kingdom are broken down. They are destroyed so that the chyme is no longer living substance or astral substance, but simple mineralised physical substance.

By simple I do not mean that its chemical structure is simple, but that it consists of physical substance, of mineralised substances only. The milk that is produced by humans and animals is not just a physical substance, but also a living and sensitive substance, although the etheric forces in it are stronger than the small trace of astrality which it carries. For this reason, Rudolf Steiner pointed out that milk, as a substance, is in the same condition as the flowers of plants; they just reach up to touch the astral forces – in the regions where the astral forces, in the words of Rudolf Steiner, kiss the flower of the plant. We find the same condition in milk.[6]

In chyme this is not the case, for it is mineralised, physical substance. Now a great deal of this chyme – I cannot give the percentage, because it is not known – is, as it were, turned into a dead substance – and this is what we excrete. In the animal it is different. Rudolf Steiner described how the 'I' which does not enter the animal itself, works in the excreted products. In humans, the substance turns away from the 'I'; it becomes dead substance. In the discussion we might consider what should really be done with it.

Now consider the mineralised chyme substance. There is no doubt that a certain amount of chyme – of this mineralised milk, this universalised substance – is now taken up through all the millions of villi of the small intestines, and carried into the lymph-capillaries which surround the intestines. Rudolf Steiner described this as follows. With our digestion we build our blood. We build the blood by lifting this chyme step by step, stage by stage, from the physical state up into the living etheric, then into the sentient, astral state, until it reaches in man a condition where it is able to carry the self-conscious 'I'. This is achieved by means of various systems that we bear within our whole organisation. Note that I do not say body; the body is only the last imprint of this organisation.

As soon as the villi have been permeated by mineralised chyme, and the lymph vessels have taken it up, it is led upwards through the thoracic tract. The thoracic tract receives all the lymph vessels from the whole lower region of the body, including the limbs; it carries the chyme up into a special vein, whence it flows into the heart. From the heart it goes upwards into our pulmonary system, where it receives through the rhythmic system the enlivening qualities of oxygen. In this way the physical chyme is lifted into the realm of living substance.

Then it is taken up by another system. At this stage, we cannot remain solely within the anatomical structure. The etheric, astral

193

and 'I' spheres are inserted into different organs, but as processes do not terminate where the physical organs do. Everything connected with the kidneys (and the cerebrospinal fluid) is a kind of physical shadow of that process which now takes up the living substance and permeates it with the forces of nitrogen, making it into sensitive substance. Then another set of processes, which are represented physically by the liver, the gall bladder and the spleen, raise it still further, so that, with the help of hydrogen, it becomes a substance which can carry an 'I'.

In this way we can see how food is taken in from above and directed from our mouth downwards where it is digested and broken down into physical matter. Then the lymph and venous blood take it upwards again. This is the second direction. Where the kidneys and cerebrospinal fluid work, a third direction comes in: this stream of substance is permeated by the forces of nitrogen from opposite sides. Lastly, the forces of the liver, spleen, and gall bladder surround the food, and with the forces of hydrogen, which work like a sheath of warmth and fire, transform it into a still higher state.

Now it is important to realise that, in a process of fire and warmth, ash falls down and light rises up.[7] The ash of the process is taken up and introduced into the brain; it is this substance that nourishes and builds up the brain. There, within our brain, we have an organ called the epiphysis or pineal gland. Once upon a time this minute, interesting and mysterious organ was in fact an eye, which looked out into the world. It was the third eye of Polyphemus, of Greek mythology. This organ receives the ash that rises up from our nutrition stream, and distributes it to the different parts of the brain. This is one process.

But there is also another process. Earlier on, I tried to show you how, wherever sensory epithelium is found, in the nose, eyes, tongue, ears and over almost all the skin, cosmic nutrition streams in, and then follows the path of the sensory nerves. All our sensory nerves are intimately connected with the brain. In the same way that the chyme goes into the large intestine to become excretion, so, as I have already described, excretion also takes place in the occipital part of the brain in the case of the optic tract; and in another part the same holds good for the acoustic tracts. But before this takes place, there is in the region of the mid-brain, in the thalamic region, a collection centre for the cosmic nutrition stream; this is the pituitary gland (or hypophysis).

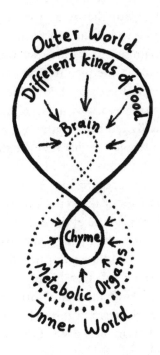

If we study the development of the pituitary gland, we find something which shows how justified it is to speak of a dividing line in the head, separating the upper from the lower part. For the pituitary gland is an organ which is derived partly from the pharynx, and partly from the brain. These two parts join together. Why? Because a centre is created there, from which the collected cosmic nutrition stream from the brain finds its way down to the organs below. This is an extremely fine and subtle process. But during the last fifty years, and especially quite recently, the pituitary gland has been found to be of utmost importance for the working of our entire organisation. It has even been called the leader, the conductor of the orchestra of our endocrine glands.[8]

The pituitary gland is intimately connected with carbohydrate metabolism, with the function of our gall bladder, with the production of milk, with the ovarian cycle in women, and with other processes involving almost the entire metabolism of our body. That certain hormones are excreted by the pituitary gland is only one side of the picture. The other side is that it is the place where the forces of the cosmic nutrition stream are collected. And if I were now to trace the different endocrine glands via the thyroid and parathyroid, right down to the adrenal glands, you would see that here are the steps whereby the cosmic nutrition stream is gradually brought down into the lower parts of our organisation. Eventually it enters the sea of lymph and the sea of the venous blood. Rudolf Steiner described, in the eighth lecture of the Agriculture Course, how hooves and nails, which are of the same material (as are, in fact, all the extreme tips of the body), are filled with substance derived from the cosmic nutrition stream.

Initially our food substances are part and parcel of the same world that we are aware of through our senses; they are outside ourselves; they are part of the outer world. Then they are taken in and gradually broken down inside our intestines. But it is important to realise that here they are still part of the outside world. The inside of the intestines is still part of the external world. Only when you pierce through the wall of the intestine are you really inside the body – in the internal world. Then the chyme becomes surrounded by our different organs, liver, spleen, kidneys, etc. Then it is lifted up, transformed, and introduced into our brain. This brain is a system that, so to speak, sticks out into the external world. It is both within and without, to the same extent that chyme is within and without.

The chyme is lifted up from the physical state and becomes a progressively living and sensitive substance. Through the forces of oxygen, then nitrogen, and finally hydrogen, it ascends to and fills and nourishes the brain as it were. Thus the whole external world streams up from below; another stream comes in through our sensory organs; it travels down in the same way that the other travels up. The existence of the cosmic and the earthly nutrition streams lies revealed in the organisation of our pineal and pituitary glands. The pineal gland receives the earthly nutrition stream from below, and the pituitary receives the cosmic nutrition stream from above and leads it downwards. There, in this very special region, the upper and the lower meet and find one another; but they must remain continually separate from one another, otherwise disease and destruction would result.

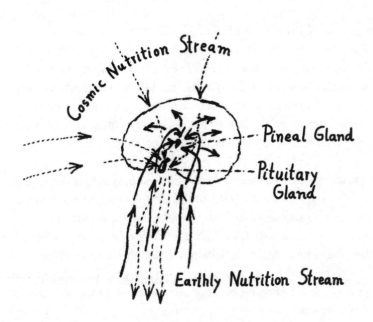

The chyme has to be lifted up through different stages, and it is this activity that creates the blood. It is not, as one usually thinks, that the chyme changes into blood substance; for the blood itself, of course, is cosmic substance. But it is the activity of overcoming the material chyme, the physical chyme fluid that keeps the blood going.

There were some questions about the difference between man and animal.
Karl König: I believe it might be possible to find a way of preparing human faeces in such a way that they can be used as manure, and need not be rejected. Usually it is said that they cannot be used, but I am not so sure. Why should it not be possible to lift this material up from its dead condition, and make it alive? Why should we not, for instance, use skimmed milk to enliven it? One would have to investigate this and give it a good deal of thought and trial. If so many synthetic materials can be made from milk, why should one not use a bit of it to enliven human compost? I can well imagine that it might be possible.

Question: What is lymph?
Karl König: It is blood without the red blood corpuscles. Lymph is entirely separate from blood. Lymph is produced more or less through the work of the spleen, the lymph glands, the thymus gland, etc., whereas the blood corpuscles have an entirely different source. Nevertheless, the sequence is quite correct: from chyme to lymph to the venous blood up to the arterial blood.

Question: Did you mean that there is a separation in the chyme between the spiritual and the physical? You spoke about it almost as if there was some ash rising. Where is the spiritual element?
Karl König: The ash rises after all this has been accomplished. But the chyme, before it has risen up and become sensitive substance and I-carrying substance, is purely physical. Out of this process, as it is a rising process, ash must fall down. And this in fact happens.

Comment: To make this comprehensible, perhaps it is necessary to imagine the chyme being lifted progressively from the physical to the etheric, the astral and the 'I' realms, when it dematerialises. When it becomes etheric it becomes like a plant juice, when it becomes astral, it becomes something like muscle tissue. If you take a piece of wood and burn it, you get warmth and a flame, which you cannot confine like a material substance, and you are left with ash. So in this process, where chyme is lifted up into higher realms, it eventually dematerialises, but some material or ash remains, and that goes to the brain.

Karl König: If you really follow the process of chyme being lifted up to living, sentient and then I-bearing substances, you will see that it is a process that occurs in a rhythmic sequence. It is like the building up of the layers of an onion, only becoming more and more delicate instead of coarser and coarser.

3 Silica and Calcium

In the last two morning lectures I have attempted to explain the cosmic and earthly nutrition streams from a particular point of view, in order now to be able to lead into a discussion of the working of calcium and silica in man, animal, plant and in the whole of nature. Let me remind you of the diagram of two intersecting lemniscates that I drew last time, indicating the cosmic and the earthly nutrition streams.

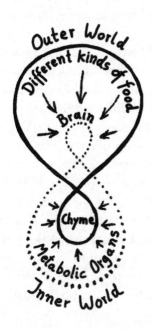

In the lower part of the upper lemniscate, chyme is formed from the substances of the outer world; the chyme is then carried up, so to speak, into the upper part of the second, the lower, lemniscate, to the head system and the brain. In the lower part of this second lemniscate our differentiated organs work together with the universalised chyme, and this is where the whole metabolism takes place.

If we take this picture of the two intersecting lemniscates seriously, it can become a key with which to unlock many of the doors hiding the wonders and riddles of existence. For no life existing here on earth can be understood without considering these upper and lower streams, and how the upper one intertwines with the lower one, and how the lower one builds up the upper one. It is a picture of the way man and the world are connected with one another. If we consider this in conjunction with what I tried to indicate with the words antipathy and sympathy, then we will gradually come to understand what nature shows us. What is important is to see everywhere how what is above creates what is below, and what is below is transformed into what is above. This is the foundation of earth existence.

During the Old Moon stage of earth evolution entirely different images and pictures would have been used; we would have had to speak about spiral figures. On the Old Sun, the teaching would again have been different. But here on earth, the lemniscate is the basic figure. It is a figure that can be used in all sorts of variations. If we can learn to transform our thinking into such forms, then we will have won the battle of thinking here on earth. We will have discovered how realities have to be thought about here on earth.

I have been told many times that it is shattering to learn that our eyes should be regarded as digestive organs. Why is this? Because if we take the image of the lemniscate seriously, we realise that in order to provide us with sense impressions, our sense organs must be digestive organs; and in order to digest our food, our liver, spleen, kidneys and intestines have to be sense organs. How can they digest if they cannot sense what they are digesting?

One of the great riddles of science today is following. when we place a substance on our tongue, how do the salivary glands 'know' exactly what kind of substance it is? The fluid they excrete changes according to the substance. Put a stone on the tongue, and nothing will flow; put meat on it, and a certain kind of saliva will be produced; for cabbage, yet another kind. But the riddle is solved if one knows that the salivary glands are not simply machines that secrete a certain amount of fluid. They secrete a particular sort of saliva because, in fact, they have tasted the nature of the substance on the tongue. In exactly the same way, our eye 'tastes' the nature and the variety of colours, and in tasting, it immediately responds by secreting a certain amount of rhodopsin for instance, with which it 'digests' the colour which it has tasted. *We* see, but our *eyes* taste. We must learn to think of our sense impressions as digestive processes, and of our nutritive and digestive processes in terms of sense impressions.

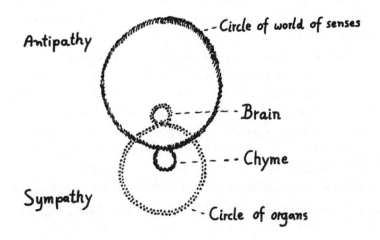

To confuse nerve-activities with sense impressions, as is often done nowadays, is of course misguided. The nerves no more sense than bones do. The liver, the spleen, the gall bladder or the kidneys can sense much more than your face can. Rudolf Steiner described in one of the lectures he gave to Waldorf Teachers in 1919, how the nerves exist simply to provide hollow spaces, and within these hollow spaces, a meeting between the self and the *maya* world of the senses can take place.[1] Nerves are a negative element in the world order, not a positive one. Nerves destroy, take away, recede.

If we understand this interplay between sense perception, digestion and nutrition, between antipathy and sympathy, between above and below, we can go one step further. We can understand how an embryo develops in the mother's womb only if we know that something descending from above joins something coming from below. It is only when the hereditary stream meets with the soul-spirit being descending onto the earth, only at the meeting place of these two streams, that the embryo is created within the sheaths of the maternal womb. The same applies to the plant. These two streams have their carriers, their bearers, their substances. The upper stream has a chariot in which to descend, and the lower stream has an escalator on which to ascend – I use these two words quite consciously (and I realise that an escalator may also go down). However, there is a chariot and an escalator that meet; these are silica and calcium.

We shall not focus on the substance itself too much, because every attempt at understanding calcium or silica from the point of view of substance is bound to fail. To explain why, I must once again call on your 'uncommon common sense', not merely your common sense. Calcium and silica must not be considered as substances, because as substances they have no value. Considering calcium and silica in exactly the same way as nitrogen, hydrogen, carbon, sulphur, phosphorus, and so on, is, as far as I can see, a big mistake.[2] Neither calcium nor silica nourishes living organisms. They do not feed plants, animals or human beings. Nevertheless, they are necessary for the whole world. We have to thank Rudolf

Steiner for so many special discoveries, but I believe that if he had pointed out only one thing, namely, how silica and calcium work in polar opposite ways in all organic as well as inorganic life, it would have served to immortalise his name and he would have to be remembered with gratitude by millions of people.

If calcium and silica are not nutrients, what are they? It is very difficult to describe what they are, but perhaps you will understand what I mean when I say that they are catalysts. They themselves do not change, but they need to be present, and in their presence all, or many, other substances start to form and arrange themselves in their proper way. We need nitrogen and oxygen as nourishment in order to build up substance. Now don't say, 'But the skeleton consists of 90% calcium.' This is true – but as calcium it has fallen out of the living stream of existence and has continually to be maintained within this living stream. You can't take bones and eat them – that is quite impossible. Nevertheless, they must be there; the shell of our skulls must be there, as must silica, in whatever form. It may be present more in the form of substance, or more in the form of an etheric force, as a process. In the first lecture of the Agriculture Course, Rudolf Steiner told us what plants would look like if only half the calcium or half the silica of the plant were there. Now understand what he means. He did not say, 'silica does this or that,' or, ' calcium does this or that,' as he did when speaking about nitrogen or oxygen. He said, 'if they were not there.'

In another lecture of the Agriculture Course he pointed to something which everyone knows who has thought imaginatively about calcium: he describes calcium as greedy. It sucks, it takes, it can't leave anything alone. The catalysing process of calcium continues until the calcium is satisfied. The more you come to understand calcium, the more you will call it *he,* like a human being. I am not saying that calcium or lime is masculine; that would give a wrong impression. But nevertheless you may call lime *he.*

In exactly the same way, if you study silica imaginatively, you will gradually come to call it *she,* as you would naturally call a ship or a car *she.* You do this because a certain affection for silica will gradually arise in your soul, and you will learn to understand that silica is not greedy at all. She too, is never satisfied and does not wish to be satisfied. She is like a highly educated person who would never stand in the way of anything, a being who has become so wise and so great that she has become nothing but a mirror for others. So here you have a *she,* but this does not mean that *'she'* is a lady. And you had the *he* who was not necessarily a man. This *he* and *she* are something much higher in creation than what is represented as male or female here on earth. It is the eternal *he* and the eternal *she* which we encounter in these substances, and this differentiation is a real necessity here. Just as here on earth the *he* is often unable to live without the *she*, and vice versa, silica can only be understood when it works together with calcium, and calcium can only be understood when it works together with silica.

A very large part of the crust of the earth consists of silica, and another large part consists of lime or calcium. Imagine what this means. Imagine that wherever we tread, the *he* and the *she* have given us the ground on which we walk; *he* because he gradually became satisfied, *she* because she gave herself up to make it possible for other substances, forces, beings, to work through and with her.

Now let us consider the human embryo. Within the uterus is the placenta, and from the placenta the umbilical cord leads into the developing embryo. The umbilical cord is one of the organs that contains the greatest percentage of silica. We can ask ourselves, why has *she* settled down, as it were, in the navel cord? What does the umbilical cord do?

The embryo is built up by cosmic forces on the one hand, and by the forces of heredity and earthly substance on the other. These two meet by means of the umbilical cord; from the placenta, the cosmic forces stream inwards, and from the embryo, the hereditary forces work outwards, and they have their meeting place in the umbilical cord; they meet in the colloidal substance of the silica sheath of this very strange and wonderful structure. In fact, this cord is an eye which looks into the cosmos on the one side, and an ear which listens to the hereditary substance on the other, to determine how much of each should meet there. What streams down from the cosmos forms itself in accordance with all that streams out of the hereditary forces.

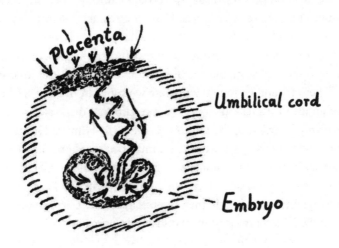

The proportion of silica in the embryo is much higher than in the child; in the child it is higher than in the adult; and in the adult it is higher than in the aged. In healthy people, between birth and death the silica content gradually decreases, while at the same time the calcium content of the body gradually rises. More and more of the silica forces from above find their way into the earthly structure, increasingly overcoming and satisfying *him*, and precipitating *him* into the body.

Superficially we can speak about silica as etheric, and calcium as astral. But in fact both calcium and silica in humans have to subject themselves to the I-organisation. Within the animal, they are subject to the astral organisation; in the plant they are subject to the etheric. So there is physical calcium and physical silica; plant calcium and plant silica. In the homeopathic *Materia Medica,* the condition in need of calcium carbonate is described as a child whose head is slightly too large, possibly tending to the appearance of hydrocephalus; the face is puffed up; the eyes are shy of light;

207

and everything runs. You recognise these people whose nose runs continually, whose saliva runs, whose ears discharge; everything looks puffy; features are not properly chiselled and hardened. This, in a homeopathic textbook, is the picture of a person who is in need of Calcarea Carbonica. In such cases, the calcium has not yet come under the forces of the 'I'; what you see is a person suffering from too much astral calcium. The astral organisation has taken up the calcium, but the 'I' has not yet inserted itself into it.

There is another condition, where we suffer from plant calcium within us. In animals, the opposite can happen – their calcium may suddenly be taken up by the forces of the 'I'. Thus, as Dr Steiner once said to Dr Kolisko, when the human being becomes ill, there is a tendency towards the animal condition; when an animal becomes ill, there is a tendency toward the human condition. These things must be understood; only then can one gradually learn to comprehend the *he* and the *she* in the world and in humans.

Now consider the inner ear. It is like a tiny *she,* inserted into the bone which lies behind our outer ear; it is entirely withdrawn from the rest of the body. The head is itself withdrawn from the body, and within the head there is an even more remote place, a place that withdraws completely. Consider this structure, and then go out into the world and observe the molluscs. If you study the formation of shells, the formation of snails, the formation of the cuttlefish, you will find in these animals exactly the same tendency that you find in the human ear – a tendency to withdraw. The shell closes itself up; the big shells require the strongest possible instruments to open them and then they immediately close again. A snail comes out of its shell – and immediately draws back again, away from the world. The cuttlefish, instead of withdrawing into a shell, surrounds itself with dark ink and swims backwards. They all, as it were, move backwards. The same tendency exists in our inner ear. All the molluscs build a shell of calcium around their body, but only because they are too sensitive; they are so much *she* that they can't do otherwise than make *he, him,* very strong. Time and again you will find calcium and silica working together in this way.

Don't think that mussels or snails are in any way typical *he* images of nature. On the contrary. This withdrawal, this 'don't touch me,' is a picture of silica. This is *she,* this is the virgin on the crystal mountain. But if *she* has to enter into life, what does she do? She takes a hard coat of *him,* of calcium, and envelops herself in it. Otherwise the equilibrium would be disturbed. Even in the plant world you find that the most tender ones have the hardest bark. Don't think that the oak is as unbending as the Teutonic people imagine it to be, not in the least. The oak is an immensely tender being. We can see Rudolf Steiner's wonderful understanding of substance when he advised us to take the oak bark and put it into the skull of an animal, where the brain would normally be.[3] It belongs there because the strong power of *him,* which is expressed in the skull bones, gives comfort and shelter to the tender existence of the oak. Is it therefore surprising that all our sense organs have, as it were, crept into our skull, and that now they sit there and just look out – the nose, the eyes, and so on? But wherever they look out, a silica sheath covers them; this is in order that the outer world can stream in. The sense organs are *she* who have looked for refuge in the place of *him,* the place of the skull.

Rudolf Steiner, in his lectures on the archangels, said that lime is not simply lime.[4] Winter calcium is different from spring calcium. In the spring, calcium starts to wake up and becomes something quite different. When the plants grow in spring, their calcium content is reduced, because they reach out to meet the sun of silica. And in the autumn, the calcium content of the plants increases again, because the plant is withdrawing down into the earth, into the hereditary stream, into digestion, into greediness. Calcium works between spring and autumn, while silica works between summer and winter.★

Although a tremendous amount of calcium is precipitated in our skeleton, the form into which it is precipitated is silica. For all those beautiful, ingeniously arranged fibres in our bones, arranged

★ This point is elaborated in the discussion following.

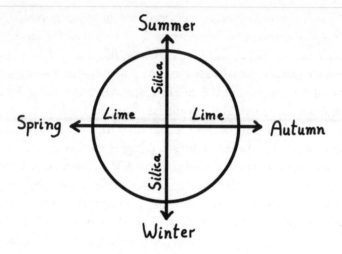

like the girders in a bridge designed by an engineer, are built by silica. When they are formed, they become filled with calcium, and the silica disappears. It recedes, and the calcium takes hold, becomes satisfied, and bone is formed. What we take as substance from the world of silica is borne on the stream of silica, and becomes chyme, which is calcium. The formation of our skull is a silica process, but its form becomes that of lime or calcium. Of course we cannot chemically change silica into calcium, or calcium into silica. We can change calcium into nitrogen, and we can change silica into an unknown substance, as Rudolf Steiner indicated in the Agriculture Course.[5] But the *he* and the *she* must always work together; silica inwards from without, gently, layer upon layer; calcium outwards from within, greedily demanding, radiating and thus filling the silica layers with calcium substance and forming shell upon shell. You should never try to gauge the forces of *him* by measuring the percentage of lime within a given organ; you might measure *her* when you find *him* as substance; because *she* uses *him* and *he* uses *her* and both belong to each other.

One thing can be a guiding principle if we try to follow the workings of calcium and silica. Wherever calcium is, there is movement; calcium and mobility are connected with one another.

Furthermore, both calcium and this mobility are subject to a higher power, to *sound*. Where there is sound and music, there is calcium and movement. For this reason, the organ of Corti (the spiral organ in the ear) is built of lime and calcium. It could not be otherwise in an organ connected with hearing. On the other hand, wherever there is silica, there is *light* and colour. Colour and light are connected with silica. Two worlds meet in the realm of substance; sound and movement, and colour and light meet, providing the basis for the existence here on earth of the soul and spirit, be they in plant, animal or the human being. Calcium and silica have enormous catalysing powers here on earth.

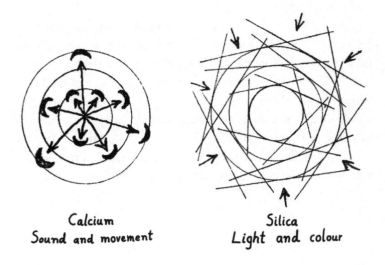

Calcium
Sound and movement

Silica
Light and colour

I have again and again tried to make the working of these two substances intelligible to our twentieth-century way of thinking. Discovering the archetypal picture of calcium and silica and living with this image for years, has helped me to understand the mysteries of these two substances.

The Gospels record a remarkable incident, where Christ was called to heal the daughter of Jairus (Luke 8:40–56). On his way to the child he suddenly stopped among the crowd, turned around, and said, 'Who has touched me?' No one admitted having done so. Then he said, 'Somebody touched me, for I perceive that power has gone out from me.' Then the woman who had suffered for twelve years from an issue of blood said, 'I did it.' While this was happening, due to the delay the girl died. Nevertheless, Christ then went and raised her. Rudolf Steiner described on several occasions how the woman and the child in fact had an intimate karmic relationship. But he also pointed to the fact that if we suffer an issue of blood, we lose calcium. Christ himself felt that forces were taken out of him; the calcium of the woman with the issue of blood caused this. Christ's own power directs the calcium within the woman's body to stay within the body and not to flow out.

The inability to hold on to substance properly is a picture of calcium.[6] Therefore, forces are taken from everywhere until the I am itself can take up the calcium and hold on to it. On the other hand, one can imagine how the twelve-year-old girl gradually withered away, because she was nothing but image, wanting to lose herself, to abandon all connection with earthly existence and to simply withdraw. But again the 'I' of the I am came and raised her, and brought her into its orbit. We may find that this picture will increasingly help when studying these two substances.

Discussion

Question: Could we hear a little more about the silica working between summer and winter, and the lime between spring and autumn? This was not quite understood.

Karl König: Just about at this time of the year, thirty years ago (in October, 1923), Rudolf Steiner described the different seasons in connection with the work of the four Archangels. There he showed us an interplay between two sets of pairs. In the fifth lecture of that course he speaks about the way – respectively – summer and winter, and spring and autumn, work together.[7] Naturally, winter turns to spring, and spring turns to summer, summer turns to autumn, and autumn turns to winter. But we must imagine that a kind of cross is inserted into the cycle of the year. At the extremities of this cross, the beings of spring, summer, winter and autumn are fixed; but further inwards, their spheres are continually changing, one into the other (see Figure on p. 210).

Lime or calcium belongs to the spring-autumn axis. Silica belongs to the summer-winter axis. Silica and calcium are catalysts of these two seasonal streams. In the summer-winter stream the cosmos streams into the earth and back again. If calcium, as the catalyst of the spring and autumn stream, were not there, the summer-winter stream would not be able to take effect. It would not be able to take hold of all the different substances, enabling them to meet, join and revolve, and then separate again. The calcium within the spring-autumn stream takes the cosmic summer-winter stream and holds it – and lets it go again. Otherwise this cosmic stream could not work in nature. For this reason the calcium content of the plant diminishes in spring, and rises in the autumn; it is like a barometer for the *she*-stream. The plant offers to all the other substances

213

a meeting place, as it were; when the meeting has taken place, it withdraws again.

Question: Does the calcium process transform into a potash and magnesium process? You say the lime diminishes in the spring. Is that because it becomes transformed into these various substances?

Karl König: I think one must look at it in the following way: calcium is especially connected with the element of iron. Silica, on the other hand, is especially connected with the element of magnesium. Now chlorophyll in plants has magnesium as its central constituent, and haemoglobin in blood has iron as its central constituent. In human beings there is the skeleton, which is, from a certain point of view, calcium; it is an accumulation of calcium. The older we grow, the more 'lime-heavy' we become. But out of the bones, blood is formed as long as we are alive. The bone marrow is the birthplace of our blood substance. Within bone marrow lies the cradle of blood, and it is the power of iron that builds it. Wherever there is calcium, iron is found too. If calcium did not have iron, the calcium would not be healed, so to speak. It is a continual healing process. In the archangel lectures mentioned earlier, Rudolf Steiner spoke of the healing influence of meteoric iron on our blood.[8] Our blood is a calcium carrier to a certain extent; we have a quantity of calcium in our blood that must continually be restrained, so that its greed, its growth and its overwhelming power are not too strong.

Silica, on the other hand, needs a consort similar to herself in nature. This substance is magnesium. Wherever magnesium appears, it creates fibres. This can be observed even in minerals. But the fibre of magnesium is not like the fibre of silica, which is transparent. In its fibrous structure, magnesium stores, so to speak, light and warmth; and then it explodes. But silica is compelled to work with the help of these forces; there is no healing process here. *He* must continually be restrained; *she* must continually be stimulated to be active. Alkalis are connected with

214

calcium, while barium, lithium and so on are connected with magnesium. It is very interesting to study geology with this in mind.

Question: Could you say something about the difference between plant silica and silica in man?

Karl König: The silica process in the human being is always located on the surface. It is found not only on the outer surface, but also on inner surfaces. Silica is distributed in our hair, all over the body in the layers of our skin where horny material is continually forming and being discarded. It is a layer in the eyes and in all the openings that form our senses. The inner and outer surfaces of the skeleton are also filled with very fine silica substance. Thus there is an outer layer of silica, and an inner layer of silica. Rudolf Steiner called this the silica scaffold of man.[9] Between these two, there is a space – and it is within this space that we develop our I-consciousness. The silica shields us from the outer as well as from the inner world. The outer world is the world around us; the inner world is the being of the blood. As conscious human beings we may not take part in either directly, but this space between the blood and the outer world is left open to us. And these two must continually be in equilibrium. In this way we can have our own, our 'private,' dream- and subconsciousness. This is the sheltering, the shielding effect of silica.

In the plant silica works quite differently. Silica forms a continuous etheric mantle around a growing plant. As in the human being iron grows within calcium, so in the plant magnesium grows within silica. Now consider a plant like equisetum (horsetail), for instance. What has this plant done? It has enveloped itself in a strong mantle of silica. It has turned physical what would normally be a kind of etheric mantle. The extent to which a plant carries silica into physical substance is an indication of its calcium power. Equisetum has a tremendous calcium power, which can be gauged by the armour of silica enveloping it. Now you can understand why equisetum plants were so huge during the Lemurian age. Lemuria represented, so to speak, a powerful attack of the *he*, of calcium, on the being of the earth. During this period huge animals developed; Rudolf Steiner once said that some of them were bigger than France is today. They swam in the soupy atmosphere of Lemuria, where also silica plants, equisetum, grew.[10] I do not know how tall they were, but I can imagine they could have been 200, 300 or even 400 feet high. A tremendous greed for power existed in the early Lemurian epoch, which had to be contained by mantles of physical silica.

Mr de Nuyl: It is of the greatest importance that to the same extent that science is developing insight into the *material* forces in matter, insight into the *spiritual* forces working in matter should be developed through spiritual science. I would like to say a few words about what science is doing with silica. Silica is used as the catalyst in the production of hydrocarbons, often together with aluminum, the clay element. Silica is used in the form of colloidal powder, which has a total inner surface of about 300 square metres per gramme or more. Now compare this to the silica preparation we use [in biodynamics]. In industry we use silica with an inner surface. And Dr Mier said yesterday that colloidal silica would not be suitable for our Preparation 501. But we use other alkaline substances, calcium and potassium; sometimes iron will work as a catalyst in the production of hydrocarbons, but only in an alkaline atmosphere. In catalysts we are working with the same forces Dr König has just been speaking about.

Karl König: This is most interesting. Colloidal silica is contained in the umbilical cord, and to an even greater extent in the lens of the eye.[11] It allows light to stream through rather than reflecting it. For years I have been struggling to understand what silica really does. In the fifth lecture of the Agriculture Course Rudolf Steiner said that silica is changed within the organism into a substance which is of the greatest importance, but which, at the moment, is not listed among the elements. Silica is transformed into this substance. What does it mean?

Question: There is an old book, Wolf's *Aschen-Analysen,* which mentions an analysis according to which a certain amount of aluminum was found in dandelions. Later researchers said that it could not be found. At the time I asked myself whether this transmuted silica might be a substance which could be mistaken for aluminum, and which might possibly have something of the nature of clay?

Karl König: You know, I could well understand this from the point of view of geology and mineralogy. Aluminum and silica are often intimately connected, and it is not clear exactly how they are held together. Perhaps there is something between the two, which so far has eluded chemical analysis. I have the impression that it must be something that is almost, but not quite, a metal, like aluminum, which is not quite a metal.

Referring to potash and dandelion, through the influence of calcium and hydrogen, potash can be created anywhere in the plant. I call this cosmic potash because it has not come via the root, but has arisen directly through the creative forces.[12]

Question: Silicas have been used in veterinary medicine for the treatment of bloating. In the light of what has been said about silica, I am wondering if instead of treating the animal after it has been attacked, one might feed silicas when there is a danger of this happening. Do you think it might be possible to develop a silica preparation for this purpose?

Karl König: I am quite certain that if we could develop a silica preparation it would work much better than silica because in silica you simply have *she,* turned into a corpse. *She* has died, and acts merely as a substance, which in the case of silica is completely inappropriate. It should not be done. One should always give silica the chance to withdraw as substance, and not to be imprisoned by it. I think that it would be much better to develop a homeopathic preparation of calcium against bloating. Then you would do justice to the nature of the cattle.[13]

4 The Endocrine Glands

Lecture 4, Sunday, October 18, 1953

Just when we have reached the point where we could really begin to deepen our understanding of substance, we have to end this course. But life is often like this, so we need not be sorry or sentimental about it.

Today we must consider, from various points of view, what Rudolf Steiner described so beautifully in the third lecture of the Agriculture Course. There he speaks about five principles: sulphur, and behind sulphur like an unseen twin, working closely with it, phosphorus; and then carbon, hydrogen, nitrogen, and oxygen. The more you read this lecture (and probably every one of you has read this lecture many times), the more you are able to imagine how these five beings actually move in a most beautiful rhythm throughout the existence of man and nature. They are mighty beings, performing a dance of creation and recreation, precipitating and dissolving substance; thanks to them each one of us, each group soul of the animals, each group soul of the plants, is able to tread the ground of this earth; thanks to them, we can work out our destinies with the group soul of the plants, the group souls of the animals, and with the earth underfoot, the throne of the world, which once was created and will last for a time. These five substances play together, perform together, on the background of silica and calcium, the *she* and the *he* of the world. They are the great catalysts, which make it possible for these five beings, sulphur and phosphorus, oxygen, nitrogen, hydrogen and carbon, to play and work together.

In 1922 Rudolf Steiner gave a series of lectures to a group of young people. He was speaking of nature, and of the laws of nature, which had been discovered during the nineteenth and twentieth centuries. And then he suddenly asked, 'Suppose nature were not, in fact, a scientist at all, but an artist?'[1] And in point of fact Rudolf Steiner said that nature was an artist. He told these young people that only by trying to live as artistically and creatively as nature herself is it possible to discover how she works. Every human being should try to do this. Rudolf Steiner quite purposely omitted a definition of carbon, hydrogen or oxygen. He does not sharply define; he does not take them and break them down; he describes and paints their deeds. Oxygen, he says, is intimately connected with all that is alive; where nitrogen is present, you will always find astral forces, but what nitrogen actually does is to lead oxygen down into the realm of carbon, where they can unite. And when you listen to such descriptions and you do not merely use your intellect, you will gradually become aware that behind Rudolf Steiner's descriptions there is an image, a real picture. The picture of nitrogen is like a being with wings, and on the wings it leads oxygen down into the physical structure of carbon. And how did Rudolf Steiner describe carbon? He called it a *schwarzer Kerl,* a 'dark customer'. At the same time he said that, although it is omnipresent, it has a hidden quality. In the Middle Ages it was called the Philosophers' Stone.

The more we study this third lecture, the more we also find that each one of these substances expresses itself in a special geometrical shape. The more we penetrate into the nature of carbon, the more we begin to realise that its forces, the way it works, its 'personality', express themselves quite objectively as a square. And we discover that nitrogen, which descends and connects oxygen with matter, expresses itself as a triangle. I only mention this in order to show how Rudolf Steiner taught. By re-reading and plunging into this lecture, by swimming in the words, we begin, as it were, to become this substance. The weight and quantity of these substances then become irrelevant, because they are omnipresent. No one can say where oxygen, for instance, appears in the body, for it appears everywhere, in proteins, fats and carbohydrates. The same applies to hydrogen. Hydrogen works in such a way that everything that has been built up is reunited again with the cosmos. Carbon is omnipresent, and so is nitrogen.

Carbon is the hidden formative power towards which all other substances are drawn. Oxygen lifts mineralised substance up into the sphere of life; nitrogen then raises it up into the realm of warmth and fire, and phosphorus carries it into the realm of light; from there, hydrogen leads it into the spirit realm.

If we understand the comings and goings of these substances, we will understand what really takes place when chyme is formed within our intestines. It is lifted up through the power of these substances step by step into living, sensitive and spiritual substance, by way of the organs that I described earlier on. The rhythmic system with the help of oxygen lifts up the chyme into living substance; the kidneys, and all that is connected with them and with the nervous system, bring about the sensitive substance; then the liver, the spleen and the gall bladder, with the forces of hydrogen, lift up what was formed in us into spiritual substance and lead it out, back into the cosmos. Imagine in this way the earthly nutrition stream, which is given up to the burning and flaming powers of the world of substance. In this burning process, ash falls out (we must imagine that it actually rises upwards), gradually reaching the brain, where it settles down; this is the bread that nourishes the brain.

On the other hand, let us consider the description of the nerves, which Rudolf Steiner gave in his lectures to physicians and priests *(Broken Vessels)*; there he describes the nerve as a digestive system. The ether, streaming in through our senses, carries light, sound and life. It travels down by way of our nerves into our entire organisation. Now we must imagine:

one stream goes out into the world, and its ash nourishes the brain; the other stream goes down into the body, furnishing us with ether substance. Rudolf Steiner described how in the sphere of our senses we actually inhale warmth; and in this inhaled warmth, light, sound and life are contained. We also exhale this warmth, but we do not exhale it into the outer world. The exhaled warmth flows into our body. In our chest system, we inhale air and exhale warmth, but the exhalation goes out not into the world, but down into our body. These two streams, the exhaled warmth, which carries light, sound and life, and the inhaled air, meet and finally settle in what science describes as lymph. This cosmic stream carries light, sound and life as it descends, and in descending it leaves the light behind in our head where it becomes our inner light. The sound is left behind to change into the inner activity of our rhythmic system. The life goes right down into physical substance, and this is what really fills and nourishes us. This life ether takes hold of carbon, the sound unites with oxygen and nitrogen, and light works together with sulphur and phosphorus.

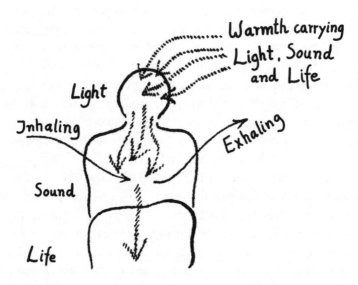

Now, where in our body do all these processes take place? As far as I can see, the key to understanding the deeds of substance, the flow of the cosmic nutrition stream, and the rising up of the earthly nutrition stream, are to be found in a series of organs which were largely neglected until about sixty years ago. These organs are the endocrine glands. The hormones that they produce are important elements in the household of the human organisation. Today, so much is known about these organs that in effect nothing is known about them any more. No one knows the beginning, the end, the middle, the top or the bottom of the subject. Nevertheless, certain facts are known about these organs, and I would now like to describe to you some of them.[2]

The day before yesterday I spoke about the pineal gland. This is the gland that receives the ash of the earthly nutrition stream from below. On the other hand, the pituitary gland receives the cosmic nutrition stream, and takes it down into our organisation. This process of exhaling warmth down into the organism is centred in this gland. If we picture how the cosmic and earthly nutrition streams work in the pituitary and

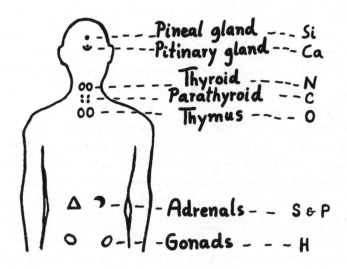

pineal glands in connection with silica and calcium, we can understand that it is the pineal gland which organises the silica structure within our body; and it is the pituitary gland which leads the calcium in and out of the body – but not in the form of earthly matter. We should not imagine that the pineal gland keeps a certain amount of silica and then spits it out wherever it is needed, or that the pituitary gland does the same with calcium.

The pineal gland is a very strange organ; in fact, it seems to manifest just the opposite of what I am saying. In the pineal gland you will find a most beautifully shaped crystalline calcium carbonate structure. Individuals in whom calcium carbonate crystals are missing from the pineal gland are what we, with our intellectual pride, have often historically called idiots or imbeciles.[3] Without these crystals, these individuals cannot place their lower 'I' effectively into the activity of their head organisation. The structure of all the silica in our organisation is held in place by this organ, in which calcium is deposited. It is the silica, the *she*, which maintains the outer and the inner sheath, as I described yesterday, whereby a space for our consciousness is formed. This is achieved with the help of the pineal gland.

If the pineal gland is damaged by disease or accident, childhood is destroyed. A three- or four-year-old child whose pineal gland is damaged changes within a few months into something like an adult person, both physically and mentally. Such a child is precipitated into matter, because silica can no longer keep the soul-spirit in a state of detachment from matter. The opposite also occurs. Where the pineal gland is too strongly at work, Down syndrome children arise – there are many such individuals today. Wherever you meet a child with Down syndrome, you know there is something about the child that is not completely individualised, but universally human.[4] Therefore such children bear a strong resemblance to each other, as if they were all brothers and sisters. They may appear to go through life untouched by earthly experience; they do not dive into sexuality and therefore their faculty to conceptualise in a 'down-to-earth' way is usually impaired. Their silica forces are so strong that the lime and calcium of the earth hardly make any impression on them. Of course, they also have a certain amount of calcium in their bodies, but their skeleton tends to be a rather soft, thin skeleton and may show some features of malformation.

Invertebrate animals are quite incapable of forming an inner skeleton. They form an outer skeleton, as it were, a silica skeleton (which in some of them, of course, becomes impregnated with calcium). Nevertheless, it is a silica skeleton. In us, this aspect of the outer skeleton is centred around the pineal gland. But the pituitary gland governs the formation of the inner skeleton. It grows out from a centre, as it were, along five radii, led down by silica. The silica-pineal complex works from without; the calcium-pituitary complex works from within. When we know this, it is no longer surprising that in some diseases of the pituitary gland the bones of the nose, the fingers and the toes suddenly start to grow. Such people develop very big hands and feet; this is called an acromegalic condition. We can see how growth is specially connected with the pituitary gland; a disorder of this gland leads either to gigantism or dwarfism. Severe dystrophic diseases of the whole skeleton like chondrodystrophia can come about if the function of the pituitary gland is compromised. Behind this gland there stands calcium. Not the earthly substance of calcium, but the inner quality of calcium, which has its seat in the pituitary gland. The being of silica, on the other hand, has its seat in the pineal gland. And between the two, the structure of our organisation is kept in form and shape. The pineal is in charge of the outer form, the pituitary of the inner form: silica and calcium: without and within, the macrocosm and the microcosm, the *she* and the *he*.

Now let us consider the thyroid gland. It lies just in front of the larynx. The thyroid gland contains a very special substance, iodine. Little vesicles within it, the thyroid vesicles, are filled with iodine bound to a special kind of protein. And what function does it serve? I will describe it very superficially to begin with. If it works too strongly, it causes a disease which you are probably familiar with, toxic goitre; gradually or suddenly, the eyes of the sufferer begin to protrude, the fingers start to tremble; the patient becomes sleepless, exceedingly restless, driven by fear and anxiety. What underlies all this is that iodine is the dark servant of nitrogen. The thyroid gland is in fact the nitrogen centre in us; but nitrogen acts by using the dark forces of iodine. It is nitrogen which astralises the whole organisation. It can do this to such an extent that people who are suffering from toxic goitre may lose twenty to thirty pounds in weight within a short time.

On the other hand, if the thyroid gland does not function strongly enough and the amount of iodine diminishes, a condition called myxoedema arises. The face of the patient becomes puffy, the skin looks inflated, and a person who was active and lively only three or four months before becomes heavy, slow, and stares aimlessly into the world; the hair falls out, and the person is sleepy and drowsy all day; every activity is slowed down. The reason for this is that nitrogen has lost its ability to carry oxygen into carbon. Therefore an enlivening process is no longer possible.

The next glandular organ is the parathyroid, four tiny little glands hidden within and behind the thyroid. These glands control the whole carbon process within our body. Only if this parathyroid is working properly does the interaction of silica and calcium in blood and bone function properly. Only then can we build a skeleton, can our blood flow. If the parathyroid is destroyed, a terrible disease, tetany, results; patients with this condition are seized with cramps because carbon asserts its formative forces too strongly, making them rigid until they die. If they were to run or exert themselves physically or mentally, they would not be able to sustain it. Children with this condition may suddenly, while at school or during a game, collapse and die instantly. They have not been able to take charge of their own oxygen.

If the thymus gland dominates in later life, you find another very strange condition. Gradually all muscular strength fades away. The muscles, as substance, remain; they are not wasted; but the patient can no longer speak or lift his hands or head.[5] Special medicines are needed to revive the muscular activity for a few hours. This is because oxygen has remained outside of the body, making it is quite impossible to bring the etheric body into the activity of the muscles. I am telling this not to shock, but to help understand and distinguish the deeper character of the different substances.

Now we come to the adrenal glands. There are two of them, and they are different from each other. The left hand one is shaped like a crescent moon, and the right hand one like a pyramid. Two substances have their seat within these glands: sulphur and phosphorus. If these glands do not function, the body more or less withers away. In the last three years, 'miracle drugs' have been discovered, which in a few hours have 'healed' rheumatoid arthritis.[6] People crippled for years received an injection, and within a few hours they were able to stand up, and attend a dance in the evening. Two days later, however, they were back in bed, and as stiff as before. What happened here? A very special substance was found in the outer part or cortex of these adrenal glands, which are situated on the top of the kidneys, and are relatively small in size. The substance that was discovered has the effect of suddenly whipping sulphur and phosphorus into action. All the sulphur and phosphorus resources in the organism are harnessed, and the human spirit can again properly take hold of his organisation. For a time, the spirit can work; it can warm and bring light into the body – but then it withdraws again. Much more could be said about these glands.

Lastly we come down to the gonads, which are the seat of hydrogen. This is the substance that connects us with the spirit.

Gathered into our body, it is the substance that leads through the generations. When the forces of hydrogen meet with the forces of sulphur (this is not intended to be understood as a chemical formula) the male being arises – no longer the *he*, but the male, descended to the earth. And when the forces of hydrogen meet with the forces of phosphorus, the female being arises. When these two meet, a child can enter the physical world again.

In this way, the pictures of the substances, which Rudolf Steiner described so beautifully in the third lecture, can become more and more comprehensible. With their help we can move from the dreamland of imagination, as it were, into the realm of destiny and human suffering. We have followed nitrogen, carbon, oxygen, sulphur, phosphorus and hydrogen in a descent that ultimately enters the hereditary stream. It is a ladder, not simply a ladder of organs, but a ladder of organs acting as the seat of the forces of these substances. A few years ago, I wrote an essay on the endocrine glands.[7] This, together with what I have been trying to say now (for instance about the diseases of the thyroid and the parathyroid glands), may help to see how nitrogen and carbon work behind the glands, so that we may find our way more and more into an understanding of substance.

The earthly nutrition stream rises up and outwards. The cosmic nutrition stream flows down the ladder of the endocrine glands, passing successively through the seats of substances, of elements, in which mighty beings weave and work within us. With this way of studying substance, we will be able to leave its purely quantitative aspect, and begin to approach the qualities of substance. Qualities can only be described in terms of real images; thus we have to describe the quality of carbon as a 'dark customer,' but we can transform this imaginary person into the square form or gesture of carbon. We can study how the bones bend when this being is unable to exert his proper strength, or what appears if he works too strongly.

What I have been trying to explain in these lectures is merely a first attempt. As I said at the beginning of this lecture, this is the stage at which we should really start, and should only be considered as an introductory lecture opening up an initial understanding of these substances. Nevertheless I am deeply grateful that you have given me the opportunity to say so many things that I have not been able to express before.

Discussion

Question: Does the crystal structure in the pineal gland alter during our life? If so, can it be harmed by the nutrition stream?

Karl König: I think this is a very important question. The pineal gland is more or less heart-shaped. The calcium carbonate crystals in it are formed like tiny little white roses; please do not take this sentimentally in any way; it is simply a fact. In a newborn child, these crystals are not present. They gradually form during the first years of childhood. They are formed by what I called the ash of the earthly nutrition stream. In later life, the whole of the pineal gland is dotted with these crystal structures, and in fact, our self-consciousness is intimately connected with them. The more conscious of our self (and this does not mean egotistical) we become, the more hardened these structures become. Although modern science regards the pineal gland as one of the endocrine glands, it has so far been unable to determine its function.

Now it can happen in childhood, in early youth or even, though rarely, in later life, that a malignant growth, a carcinoma, develops in this gland. In adults, this causes a change of consciousness. In children, you find what I described earlier, a condition called macrogenitosomia praecox. I once saw a four-year-old girl who, through an unfortunate accident, had run a splinter through her eye into her skull right into the pineal gland which was destroyed. I saw her a few months after this accident; she was four-and-a-half years old. Her breasts were already developed, she had started to menstruate, and she had grasped all sorts of mathematical and arithmetical calculations within a few weeks. Her intellectual thinking had suddenly awakened. The child with Down syndrome, on the other hand, has great difficulty grasping numeracy. These children can repeat 'one and one is two,' and they can learn to say 'one, two, three, four, five,' but without actually being able to add up or count in a meaningful way.

When you study the psychology of children with Down syndrome, it is most striking to see that not only do they not have any real connection with sexuality, but they have no connection with death either. The problem of death, which is so clearly present for every normal child, however young, does not exist for the child with Down syndrome. Even when they grow up, turn eleven, twelve, thirteen, they remain utterly indifferent to death. It is also one of the most difficult educational tasks to awaken in them a religious experience. They are, however, very good mixers. If a child with Down syndrome mixes with other children, the atmosphere is typically happy and light-hearted. They are the *she*, which does not touch, but arranges everything. Therefore they are also much better able to imitate than other children. Their skin tends to be considerably harder than that of other children; they develop a kind of outer skeleton, because the structural forces of their inner skeleton are so compromised.

Question: Can you link food grown with chemical fertilisers to the question of consciousness, and also the question of morality?

Karl König: I am very glad you have brought up this question. I believe we must become much clearer about the implications of food grown with chemical fertilisers. What I have to say now is a purely personal idea: I have, as yet, no proof of this, but somehow it is a personal conviction. As far as I can see, when we eat chemically fertilised food, it does not nourish us, because the processes described as the earthly nutrition stream entirely dissolve it and leave no ash behind to feed the brain. We dissolve it all back into the spirit, so that it can be taken up and 'rebuilt.' Properly grown food is more earthly. Artificially grown food is not more earthly, it is more spiritual, but in the wrong way. And as a result, is does not leave any usable ash behind. Organic food and biodynamic food leave enough ash to keep our I-consciousness awake and in existence. With eating this food, people become too spiritual, but in the wrong sense. I am convinced that if we go on eating only this kind of food we will revert to a dreamlike condition. We will fall asleep, we will not be able to keep awake; we may even revert to previous states of consciousness, possibly even imagining things of wondrous beauty, but our self-consciousness, which connects us with the being of Michael, will not be able to establish itself. This is how I see it. Artificially based agricultural methods affect our mental condition much more than our physical condition. The body can be fed easily, because it is built up by the cosmic nutrition stream. But feeding the brain is our own responsibility.

Question: Has what you have just been saying something to do with the statement of Dr Steiner, I think in 1905 or 1906, that in the future our food will become more and more mineral?
Karl König: That is so. We shall take in food that does not feed anything but the brain. Rudolf Steiner spoke about this as a future form of appropriate nutrition. But by the 'future' he meant many, many hundreds of years hence.

Question: At present, salt is the only mineral we eat. Is that, so to speak, the first seed? When one follows up historically how people used to season their food, one finds that they used relatively little salt.
Karl König: In bread you take in a great amount of minerals. Not only as actual salt. Actually, it is bread that must gradually become the mineralised food. Bread will have to turn into salt.

Question: It is not that we shall have to live on the minerals as we find them in nature, but that we ourselves shall have to produce them?

Karl König: On the other hand, through our cosmic nutrition stream, many minerals come in – especially metals. Rudolf Steiner once described how, for instance, copper is taken in through the ears, tin is taken in through the eyes, and so on. These are all minerals.

Comment: I think it is quite an important point that the biodynamic method is not a more ethereal, but a more physical one. Rudolf Steiner said that through the use of chemical fertilisers the plant lives practically only in the realm of water, and withdraws from the realm of the earth, from the solid realm. One of the main functions of the biodynamic method is to bring the plant into a more profound contact with the mineral forces of the earth. I see the Agricultural Course as the first step on the road to the right mineralisation of food. I do not think Dr Steiner meant that in the future we should grind up granite and make food out of it, but that we should strengthen the natural mineralising processes.

Question: Would you say something about the calcium supplements produced by Weleda?
Karl König: Calcium supplements were indicated by Dr Steiner after the First World War for undernourished children in Germany and other parts of Central Europe. What is malnutrition? It occurs when the spirit cannot take hold of the body, when the pituitary gland has lost its power to connect the upper stream, the cosmic nutrition stream, with the body. To stimulate the cosmic nutrition stream in the body, carbonate and phosphate of lime are given in the form of calcium carbonate and apatite.

Question: How could one look upon the nourishment of animals with artificially grown food, which is increasingly being used nowadays? The picture would look different, would it not?
Karl König: I do not think it is so very different, if you put

dream-consciousness in the place of I-consciousness. Rudolf Steiner again and again emphasised that cattle must be allowed to go outside and use their sense of smell. What is thinking in us, in animals is smell. And this artificial food reduces the 'smelliness' of the food, so that the cattle lose their ability to discriminate when they are finally let out.

Question: If the biodynamic method is the more physical one, could you explain why Rudolf Steiner said that if you use chemical fertilisers, they should first be put through the compost heap? *Karl König:* That is right. In the compost heap they receive something. They are not lifted up, but pulled down, connected with the earth. You see, what I have described as the cosmic and the earthly nutrition streams are really a kind of curtain, which conceals something behind it. If you pull back this curtain, you come to the secret, to the inner cell, so to speak. You come, on the one hand, to the brain, and on the other hand, to the lymph. In the brain, behind the curtain of the cosmic and the earthly nutrition streams, there rests our past karma. In the lymph, there rests our future karma. If we do not properly unite ourselves with these two focal areas of karma, we will have no proper connection with either our past or our future.

Behind all that I have described stands this picture: physically, we bring our heredity with us. Spiritually, we bring our past karma with us. It streams down into our limbs, and makes us do what we have to do, makes us go to the places where we have to go, and meet the people we have to meet. But at the same time, our future karma is already beginning to manifest within us. Wherever our lymph flows, it is leading us on into our next life. We live between our future and our past karma. There are some very severe diseases of the lymph. Suddenly the lymphocytes start to increase; it is my impression that this frequently happens in human beings when they struggle to establish a relationship with their present karma. Then their future karma starts to rise up, and what would be appropriate for the next life turns into disease in this life. It is not surprising, for instance, that the great poet Rilke, who never fully arrived on the earth, died of such a disease.[8] This illness is becoming more and more prevalent in our time.

Question: If the pineal gland is the seat of self-consciousness, why does consciousness apparently become so bright when it is destroyed?
Karl König: It is the intellect, not consciousness, which becomes so much clearer.

Comment: The pineal gland in reptiles is very well developed.
Karl König: Very well developed indeed. It is a beautiful organ in some of them, in the lizards, for instance. There it is still a functional eye. If you follow the development of the pineal gland, it starts as a kind of eye, sticking out like a lamp. It is an eye that does not see light, but senses warmth. It is an organ of warmth. In the course of evolution, it has become smaller and smaller and now it is a minute structure. Through the warmth which it received, the great imaginations, or mythological pictures, streamed in. This died out, the head closed; the skull, with the cortex, shut down the clairvoyant powers, which the pineal gland gave us. So we became thinkers instead of clairvoyants. This is inscribed in our bodies, and our body is the script of the evolution of the world. You can read this script if you are able to decipher its letters. A textbook exists in which all the different pineal glands of all the species of animals are described.[9] It is most interesting.

Es ist also das Folgende zu beachten!

Die Nahrung, die durch den Mund aufgenommen wird, wird _verallgemeinert_. Sie wird generalisierte Substanz; Chymus, das eigentlich _Milch_ ist. Dann wird dieser Keim neu gebildet.

Es ist also der Verdauungsprozess ein _umgekehrter_ Embryonalprozess, er _entbildet_, das, was gebildet war; führt es zurück zum _Keim_. Dieser Keim wird nun durchätherisiert, astralisiert + durch-icht. (Das tun die drei Systeme: Lunge-Herz, Niere, Galle-Milz.) Das, was da gebildet wird strömt z.T. zurück in die Welt (Atmung,) z.T. hinauf in das Gehirn s wird dort abgelagert.

Dem gegenüber steht der Kosmische Ernährungsstrom. Er geht ein durch die Sinnesorgane s bleibt ein durchaus Vielfältiges, Uneinheitliches. Dieses Un-Einheitliche, Mannigfaltige befruchtet dauernd mit ätherischer Kraft den Keim der Lymphe. Daraus wird aber immer neu der Leib des Menschen entwickelt s d.h. gebildet.

Haupt: Kosmische Form + physische Substanz
Glieder: Physische Form + Kosmische Substanz.

From Karl König's notes for a lecture in Stuttgart,
November 3, 1953, on the process of the cosmic nutrition stream.
There is no transcript of this lecture.

The following needs to be born in mind:

Food taken in through the mouth
is <u>universalised</u>, turned into generalised
substance; chyme, which is actually milk. Then
this germ is created anew.

This means that the digestion process is a <u>reversed</u>
embryonic process, it <u>de</u>-forms what has been formed,
leading it back to the <u>germ</u>. This germ is then
etherised, astralised and permeated by the forces of the 'I'. (This is
effected by the three systems: lung–heart, kidney, gall bladder–spleen.)
Part of what is created through this process streams back into the
world (breathing); another part streams up into the brain and is
deposited there.

Over against this there is the cosmic nutrition
stream. It streams in through the sense organs
and retains its manifoldness; it is not homogeneous.
This non-homogeneous, manifold process
continuously fertilises with etheric power the germ of the lymph.
From this the human body is continually
developed anew, i.e. built up.

Head: cosmic form and physical substance
Limbs: physical form and cosmic substance

The Meteorological Organs

Six lectures for farmers at Botton Hall, Yorkshire, October 30 to November 3, 1958

1 Introduction

Lecture 1, Thursday, October 30, 1958

It is not only a great pleasure for me to be able to give these lectures, but it is an honour to speak as a medical doctor in a circle of farmers and gardeners about such spiritual subjects as we are going to discuss during the next few days. I think the last time I was asked to speak in this circle turned out to be a momentous event for all of us. We were somehow able to identify our common striving to understand the subject in hand. When Mr Wood approached me I was grateful for the opportunity to speak once again for a few hours, and to work with you during these days on this very important subject of the meteorological organs of man.[1]

You will understand that I am not just going to hold lectures; I would be very grateful if we could become a study group in which we will really try our best to arrive at a deeper understanding of some of the indications which Rudolf Steiner gave to doctors on the one hand, and to farmers on the other hand. During the last three years, several hundred doctors working together in the Anthroposophic Medical Association in Stuttgart have been discussing this very special theme. Our recent conferences in Germany dealt precisely with the theme of the four meteorological organs in connection with human metabolism, focusing particularly on protein formation in the human organism. I cannot say that we have reached any conclusions, nor that we have solved some of the main problems. We have tried, however, to gather together certain facts which surprisingly have been ignored by modern science during the last fifteen or twenty years. During the course of these conferences, I had often felt that it would be necessary to bring some of these facts to the attention of biodynamic farmers. The invitation to speak to you again therefore coincided with my own intentions. This is why we are here now, and I hope that it will be a fruitful exploration for all of us.

I would like to make clear at the outset that everything I am going to present to you is, of course, based on the indications of Rudolf Steiner, as well as upon what has been elaborated during the last three years amongst these doctors. Therefore I would like you to be aware of the fact I am not claiming sole credit for many of the things I am going to say. Many doctors have been involved in piecing things together, and I am quite unable to attribute any of them to particular individuals, as I would not be able to remember the specific details – so behind what I am going to say there stands the work of the German Anthroposophic Medical Association.

This evening I would like to give a kind of overview of the whole subject we are going to be discussing in more detail later. I would like to speak about the human being in general as he appears in front of us, as we appear to ourselves. Of course, only a mere fraction of what the human being really is presents itself to our own awareness either as individuals or as members of a social organism. First of all we have our daily experience. We look into the world; we can see and hear with our senses, touch, taste and smell. We fill all these sensory experiences with our thoughts and ideas. We build up certain images of the world. We experience feelings; we act by means of our volition. All this we *do*. All this we *are;* all this is something we also encounter in meeting other human beings. Yet it merely constitutes the surface of everything that we are.

This fraction of the human being is the one to which we usually refer when we as students of anthroposophy describe the human being who can think, feel and exercise will. We ascribe to this being, with regard to the physical and etheric makeup, a sense-nerve system, a rhythmic system and a metabolic-limb system. But again, this is no more than a superficial view.

While this classification provides a fundamental insight into the superficial nature of the human being, behind, underneath and above it, there is much more to discover. Human words are barely able to describe it. Behind this surface appearance is the true and actual being of man. Our own theories and constructs fall short when – as sometimes we are able to do with a sense for the true reality of the human being – we encounter something with which we are totally unfamiliar. We may meet someone who has suddenly lost his rational consciousness, who starts speaking in incomprehensible sentences, disclosing certain things that are totally alien to us, and we wonder what has happened to this person. Then, in order to defend ourselves and in order to maintain our own identity, we label them insane. We classify them in a way that enables us to free ourselves from the impact of such an experience, so that we will not be overwhelmed by what is coming towards us.

Yet here we meet something that is much more real, much closer to true human existence, than that which normally speaks to us through the *maya* of surface appearances. This is an ailment intimately related to what we are going to discuss during the next few days.

In this context I should like to refer to a lecture by Rudolf Steiner where he describes what happens when the human being is gradually approaching the end of pre-earthly existence.[2] He said that the spiritual beings, the beings of the higher hierarchies have intuitions. The results of these intuitions are the physical organs of the human body, the major organs such as the liver, spleen, kidneys, heart and lungs.

We hardly experience these organs as part of ourselves, insofar as our awareness is confined to our waking existence and rational consciousness. They belong to a realm that is much more general, in no way personal or individual. They are still part of the gods, almost as if the gods had their sense organs within us, in our body.

This is what we have to become aware of. First of all, we should learn to see that these organs no longer form part of human individuality or of the personality. They are much larger, much more all-embracing than is, for instance, our skin or our nervous system.

Some of you will have heard of the famous and great zoologist and thinker, Professor Portmann of Basle University.[3] In recent years he has tried to introduce a new and, I think, significant idea, which is closely linked to what I have just tried to express. Portmann has drawn our attention to the fact that in the animal kingdom the individuality of a species expresses itself on the surface, but not internally. If you remove the skin from both a lion and a tiger, and you examine the two carcasses, you will no longer be able to tell one from the other. It is virtually impossible. What is underneath the skin of the tiger is almost exactly the same as what is underneath the skin of the lion. He says that the same thing can be observed in many other cases. He draws attention to the fact that the nature of the surface is connected with the all-embracing power of light. The light creates the individuality. (When I say individuality, I am referring to the group soul of the particular species.)

In the case of the human being the situation is quite different. In the structure of our nose, in the way our hair grows, the way our wrinkles are formed and the lines of our hands are drawn, in the way everything expresses itself outwardly, we find the deep expression of our individual existence, of our personality. If, however, we go a little deeper, if, for instance, we study the major organs, we are no longer able to discern any kind of individuality. Rather, the organs are formed and shaped by all that surrounds us: The landscape, the geological formation of the earth, the constitution of the water, the climate, all these factors build, shape and give form the major organs.

I can well imagine that a few centuries from now, when we

will have gained greater insight into all these questions, we shall be able to say the following: externally, human beings expresses themselves as individuals, but in everything that comprises the lung, the heart, the kidney and so on, they express the life that the entire existence encompassing heaven and earth has bestowed on them in accordance with their individual karma. From a medical point of view, and also if we really want to understand human existence, we must come to the conclusion that everything connected with so-called mental illnesses is based on a physical and etheric disturbance of what is general in us.

Psychotic patients during the acute phase of their condition – I don't say illness – lose their personality. They are no longer their individual self. Something general, something universal, something cosmic is coming to expression through them. Perhaps it is the voice of the liver that sounds through them; the voice of the liver is the voice of many spiritual beings who have worked together in the intuition to create this organ, and the human being is merely the mouthpiece for this.

Please do not misunderstand me by thinking that individuals in this condition are thereby superior or better than we are. I am not making any judgment here. I am only describing how our individual illnesses are connected with the individuality, the spirit, whose task it is to live in this body, which is formed in a general and universal way, to live as an individuality in what the universal beings – the formative powers of the cosmos – have given to us.

The above remarks may serve as a kind of introduction to what I want to say.

I would now like to draw your attention to the four major organs – or organ systems – that Rudolf Steiner presented to us in so many different ways and from so many different perspectives. His different descriptions sometimes appear to contain contradictions; he left it to us to work through these contradictions and in so doing find out what he really meant.

The way he spoke about the heart and its activity is of

particular interest. He described how the pathological activity of the heart is not connected solely with the individuality. The heart depends on the active mobility of the human being himself. Rudolf Steiner described how the function of the heart suffers if the active mobility of human being is restricted, and speed determined from outside is imposed on them. Remember that Rudolf Steiner said this as early as 1920, and realise how much more significance and impact his observations have for our own time, almost thirty years later.

Imagine sitting in a car, either driving or being driven, or travelling in an aeroplane, being exposed to speeds of 100, 300, 400 miles an hour or more. We do not actively achieve this speed, but we are forced – there is no other way of putting it – to suffer this speed. The whole human warmth organisation, with the heart at its centre, is restricted as a result, because it is dependent on warmth (mobility) from outside. Our active mobility no longer creates its own warmth if we don't walk or use our arms and hands. If we sit, we do not produce any active warmth, but are dependent on warmth from outside.

Nevertheless, the speed is a reality, as is also the activity of the heart. Just imagine that when we are walking, our heart beats quite differently from how it beats when we are sitting down. When we are climbing, our heart's activity is entirely different from its activity when we are just walking on level ground. On the other hand, if we rise a few thousand feet into the air, and the heart remains seated, as it were, or if we rush through the countryside but aren't actually moving, the whole of the warmth organisation reflects irregularities back to the heart.

Rudolf Steiner once said, 'It is necessary for people who suffer from heart disease to always have a certain amount of active movement.'[4] No wonder that today the majority of deaths are due to heart problems. We are no longer using our limbs, and the heart is the organ that suffers as a result. This is the first point. I don't want us to draw any conclusions at this stage; I am simply putting facts before you. You can see what Rudolf Steiner meant by a meteorological organ when he speaks of the heart in connection with speed. It concerns not only the heart's relation to atmosphere or thunderstorms, to rain or anything like that, but also to the individual or passive speed.

From this particular point of view the second organ – the bladder – is even more interesting. In this particular context Rudolf Steiner did not mention the kidneys, but one gets the impression that he treated the bladder as representative of the entire urinary system.

He described the bladder as a hollow organ that sucks. It continually sucks that which is not able to suck. The bladder in fact sucks our whole breath. This might seem very strange to you, yet it is so. We do not breathe with our lungs. Although the air streams into our lungs, the process of breathing is continually carried out by the activity of this organ, the bladder. Out of the gaseous elements in the blood, urine is formed, and the fluid drops down continually and very rhythmically, while the process itself is regulated by the active sucking action of the bladder. Like the rhythmical beat of the heart, the sucking activity of the bladder is disturbed by the outer activity of our movements, by the mobility of our arms and legs, but most of all it is disturbed by what Rudolf Steiner called *innere Beweglichkeit,* inner mobility.

How did Rudolf Steiner describe this inner mobility? He pointed out, for instance, that if we do not sit down to eat and chew properly, but rather gulp our food down, then our inner mobility is disturbed. Then the muscles of our pharynx, our stomach and our duodenum, of our whole intestinal tract, are moving restlessly and much too quickly, resulting in a permanent inner tension, a continuous restless inner activity.

Although he did not mention it, it is quite obvious that the outer activity is performed by the striated, voluntary muscles, while the inner mobility is generated by the involuntary muscles, those muscles that are found in our intestinal tract and in almost every internal organ. Through our restlessness, the rhythmical sucking activity of the bladder is disturbed. The process of breathing is disturbed, and as a result the whole of the interaction between the astral and 'I' on the one hand, and the physical-etheric on the other hand, is thrown out of gear. We are able to observe precisely the very subtle differences arising in such circumstances.

The third organ that Rudolf Steiner described is the liver. In the liver we already find ourselves, as it were, 'outside' of the compound of the human body. Rudolf Steiner described the liver as a kind of inner mirror of the condition of the water in the region where we live – whether this water contains a greater or lesser amount of lime, or silica, or whatever. This is mirrored in the activity and condition of the liver.

The fourth organ is the lung. Now we are moving still further towards the outside of the body, because the lung and everything connected with breathing is related to the whole surrounding world around us, not only to the air itself, but to the whole geology of the earth. Studying the geology of a certain region is the same as studying the lungs of the inhabitants of that region. Here we are really dealing with an opening out process, whereas in the liver we have a kind of narrowing process. The bladder is confined to our inner mobility, whereas with the heart, the world remains entirely outside. These are facts that we shall have to consider in more detail in the course of our deliberations.

In another context, Rudolf Steiner approached these same four organs from an entirely different angle. At this stage I am merely trying to gather descriptions together. He described how, within us, these four organs constitute areas where something belonging to the structure of the whole earth is repeated.

We have the physical ground of the earth surrounded by the hydrosphere and the atmosphere. According to Rudolf Steiner, the atmosphere is surrounded by a layer or sphere of warmth. Above this sphere of warmth there is the sphere of light. He then said something that I can only relate, but which I feel is of the utmost importance for our time. He stated that in this sphere light 'grows'; light is actually created. He used the term as we would when we speak of plants *growing* here on earth. Here light is growing, which means that original light is streaming down to the earth, but not from the sun. Beyond this stream of light there is a sphere that he called 'genuine chemistry', and beyond that again there is a sphere of vitality, of the life ether.

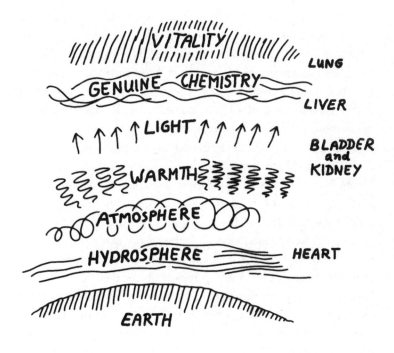

Then Rudolf Steiner pointed out that we also carry these spheres within us, where we create warmth, original light and genuine chemical forces, and where we have to insert this tremendous vitality into the one organism in a balanced way. Out of these arise the heart, the bladder – again in conjunction with the kidneys – the liver and the lung.

What is around the earth is inverted into our own body and appears as the heart organ, the kidney organ, the organs of lung and liver. Rudolf Steiner then said the following: these four organ systems are the actual creators of the substance albumen.

Regarding the transit of substances through the intestinal wall, various statements have been made. Experiments in humans using radioactive markers such as a 'harmless' carbon isotope, have been used. These elements subsequently show up in different organs. The persorption[5] rate of various toxic substances, such as DDT, is also known. This rate is even higher in infants than in adults. However, albumen is continually being created – I cannot say in our body, that would not be quite true – but rather within the *system* of our existence.[6] The four focal points – liver, lung, heart and kidney – tell us about the intuitions of the spiritual beings around them. A continuous process of forming and dissolving is taking place. The heart supplies to this process of albumen formation the element of hydrogen, the kidney supplies oxygen, the liver nitrogen, and the lung carbon.

We must call to mind the description Rudolf Steiner gave before the Christmas Foundation Meeting, on December 1, 1923, about the coming into being of the earth.[7] He described how in the early Lemurian epoch – probably the first and second periods of the Lemurian epoch – the whole earth was not surrounded by, but consisted of, an atmosphere of albumen. If we take this statement seriously, it means that at that time it would have been quite impossible to distinguish the five elements or substances – carbon, hydrogen, oxygen, sulphur, nitrogen – because they did not yet exist then. What was present was a higher substance: albumen.

Let us recall some of this description: how plant beings suddenly appeared and disappeared like clouds; how, under the influence of cosmic life, parts of the albumin coagulated, forming small clots; how there was a rain of lime which filled these forms of clotted albumen, resulting in the first animals, which began to appear in the life of the earth. We must imagine this as vividly as possible and try to understand how this sphere of albumen – this higher substance – gradually condensed, becoming the hydrosphere, the atmosphere, and finally the hard physical core of the earth. We must imagine how these spheres gradually rose up, making possible the processes of differentiation; how, out of the air which became clear, light grew; how out of the hydrosphere, chemistry or chemical ether arose, and how, as a counterforce to the physical condensation, the original vitality, the life ether, spread its mantle around this planet. If we see how, out of this original unity, the seven spheres gradually developed and formed themselves, we begin to understand how the human being gradually made himself at home in his physical body.

In describing this, Rudolf Steiner pointed out that we feel intimately connected with all this. It is as if we were able to remember our own childhood. It is like an experience in our childhood, which later rises up in us again so that we remember it. Because we were part of all that has happened in the course of creation, it belongs to us and comes back to us during the course of our life. It is this memory to which Rudolf Steiner called our attention; it is our own memory that we are speaking about.

This gives us a much more intimate understanding of how the process of albumen or protein formation within us is only a miniature counterpart of what was present for the whole earth at the beginning of Lemuria. This we carry within us as a kind of living memory. Spiritual beings are working within this continuous process of protein formation. Spiritual beings play a role within our existence. The whole cosmos permeates our own individual existence: the outer space becomes an inner space. Throughout all meteorological conditions these organs reach far beyond space and time. Yet, inasmuch as we are a *body,* they exist within us. They relate us to the cosmos as long as we do not destroy them completely in their rhythm, for instance by destroying the activity of our heart or the activity of our bladder.

If in addition we cut ourselves off from the living flow of the water, from the proper influence of the soil and the earth, we will no longer correspond to our own picture of ourselves. We will be nothing but a shadow or spectre of what was once alive in man.

Nowadays things are much more serious than ever before. We know that whenever we are speaking together about such influences and such ideas, it is not only ourselves who are involved when we think; we are also enlightening the spiritual surrounding of at least part of humankind by our thinking.

So far we have approached our topic in general terms. Tomorrow we shall begin to go into details. I should like to begin by speaking about the system of the lung to enable us to understand the nature of the lung in the context outlined today.

2 The Lung

Lecture 2, Friday, October 31, 1958

Today we shall venture into the territory of the four great organ systems. It is from these that the albumen or protein constituting the main substance of the human body is really created; it is continually being created anew and simultaneously dissolved. Sometimes, when I try to enter this region in thought (of course this is only possible with the help of Rudolf Steiner), I find myself being led to the following picture: this region resembles the one described by Goethe in his *Fairy Tale of the Green Snake and the Beautiful Lily*. The Green Snake enters the underground cave for the first time, radiant light emanating from her body due to her having swallowed gold coins dropped by the Will 'o the Wisps. There she encounters the figures of the four kings. It is dark, and the light from her body is just sufficient to enable her to make out the figures of the Gold and Silver Kings. Then the Old Man with the Lamp appears, and the figures of all four kings emerge more clearly.

This is the kind of image that can guide us time and again. It is virtually impossible to approach the reality of these four organ systems in an intellectual way. We must use imaginations – imaginations we have been given by great seers such as Goethe, Rudolf Steiner and others. Eventually such images may help us to come closer to an understanding of what we are searching for.

I would also like to remind you of something that Rudolf Steiner once mentioned to doctors. Referring to proteins, he made a fundamental distinction between the two forms of protein – one of them constituting the substance of plants, and the other providing the basis for the ensouled nature of animals.[1] He made it clear that these two forms of protein are incompatible with each other. Animal protein, especially human protein, is destroyed, so to speak, when plant protein comes close to it, and vice versa. They are incompatible even though chemically plant protein consists of exactly the same substance as animal and human protein.

Then he added something that we should take as a kind of image. Animal (and especially human) protein is created not by the four organ systems, not by the organs themselves. So whenever here I refer to organs, I always mean the systems. Imagine the sphere of human protein.

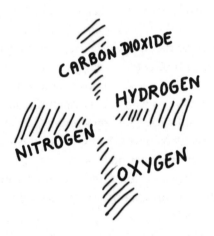

These huge systems of lung, liver, heart and kidney, along with the bladder, are the creators of human protein. Plant protein is not created by these four 'guardians' that the spirit has inserted into us, but through the agency of carbon, hydrogen, oxygen and nitrogen. Plant protein is created directly by the building powers of these substances. The forces that are working directly in the plant take on another form in the human organism. The cosmic powers of carbon turn into the lung system. A corresponding relationship exists for the other three. If we were to describe this as an image, we could say that they become kings. The cosmic powers do not manifest directly, but in disguise. In this metamorphosis these cosmic powers create the protein within the human frame. This is a kind of introduction to what we will now try to elaborate in greater detail.

Let us now turn to the organ system of the lung. We are all familiar with the lung. We also know a certain amount about its form and about its function. We know that the organ of the lung is, at least according to our superficial understanding, the organ of breathing. Yet Rudolf Steiner repeatedly spoke about the lung as an organ whose function of taking in air is merely a sideline that facilitates the exchange between air, light, oxygen and carbon dioxide.

In its essential reality or nature the lung is something quite different. In my overview last night, I mentioned that the lung is especially connected with the element of earth rather than the element of air. Rudolf Steiner indicated that as a meteorological organ the lung is intimately related to the structure of the soil in the area where we live. In fact, studying the geology of an area is equivalent to studying the lungs of the people in that region.

How is this to be understood? If we study the anatomy of the lung, we find that in the very early developmental stages of both humans and animals, the primitive lung grows or buds out of the intestinal tract. This in itself poses a big question. Why does the lung – an organ of breathing which belongs intimately to our rhythmic system – originate in the intestinal tract? Why is its source of existence related to the organs of the metabolic system? For the moment, I will leave this as an open question.

The lung develops in a way that can be described as a continuous budding process, always budding in pairs. This constitutes a dichotomic process of development, which is a very plantlike process. It is as if a plant were growing and dividing, and again dividing, and dividing again. One can speak of a stem and branches. From the branches the twigs arise, always two at a time, and you can imagine that in this way the whole of what is quite appropriately called the bronchial tree with its branches develops.

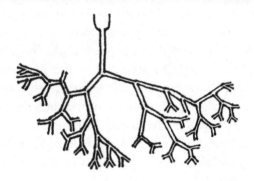

At the ends of this bronchial tree, in the ends of millions and billions of these tiny twigs, the tiny air sacs or alveoli are to be found. Within these vesicles the exchange between oxygen and carbon dioxide takes place. Each one of these vesicles is surrounded by a network of blood capillaries. You must imagine that the surface of the blood capillaries, as well as the constitution of the alveoli, is extremely delicate. It consists of an exceedingly thin film, like a layer of fine gauze. Through this film, oxygen streams in and carbon dioxide leaves in a process of exchange.

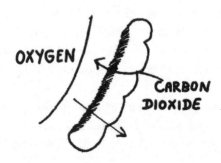

How does this exchange actually take place? Physical laws at present do not appear to be able to account for it, but imagine the enormous surface area of those millions of alveoli. If I remember rightly, someone once estimated that their surface area, which unfolds within the thoracic cavity, is equivalent to the surface area of Lake Geneva or Lake Constance. Be that as it may, it is certainly very large. Across this extensive surface within us, the exchange of gases takes place.

Nevertheless the lung in its early embryonic stages appears to be destined to become a gland similar to, for example, a salivary gland. However, its potential to develop in this direction is diverted. It becomes instead hollow and empty, to allow the air to stream in. It is as though its generative function as a gland had sacrificed itself. Instead, it develops a potential for inner space. This confers on the lung a somewhat dubious status. Its destiny was to become a gland, but this changes. It originates from the intestinal system, but both its structure and function are diverted away from the intestinal tract. Is it possible, I wonder, to fathom, the character of the lung as an organ? Is it possible to discover and to understand its essential nature?

In studying the anatomy of many fish, we find something like a lung, situated roughly as shown in this sketch. However, it is filled with air, but *not from outside*. It is in fact an air bladder, which in the fish produces its own air. Air actually issues into this bladder continually. As you can see here, the lung reveals its inner nature as an air gland. We are familiar with glands that produce fluids, but the lung is a gland that at a certain stage in its evolution produced air.

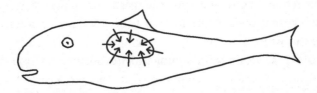

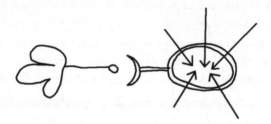

The production and dissolution of air within this glandular lung, in this air bladder, is a continuous process. We can begin to discover its essential nature if we consider that this air bladder is connected with a set of tiny bones. These are ossicles, comparable to the ones that connect the eardrum in the middle ear to the inner ear. These little ossicles reach up to the vestibular organ, the organ of the three semi-circular canals.

Through this organ, which is more or less fully developed in fish, the fish maintains its balance with respect to its activity in its surroundings. The air bladder becomes smaller or larger, continually influencing the fluid dynamics within the three semi-circular canals and thereby regulating the fish's balance as it swims and floats.

Now recall how Rudolf Steiner described the being of the fish in those wonderful lectures that he gave in 1923 about the nature of animals.[2] Speaking about the nature of fish, he says that fish have a kind of consciousness for the whole ether structure of the globe. Fish swim within the whole ether sphere of the earth and (although these are not exactly Rudolf Steiner's own words) fish have to maintain their balance within the structure of the whole of three-dimensional space. The air-gland-bladder, which corresponds to the lung in fish, is intimately connected with this process.

Earlier we described the lung as an organ that has sacrificed its glandular nature, its ability to create its own air, so that the air from outside can stream in. Now remember Rudolf Steiner's description of the urinary bladder as a sucking organ, an organ that, because it is a hollow organ, is endowed with the ability to suck. Related to this organ is the lung-bladder, whose structure, in the case of fish, should be pictured as in the drawing.

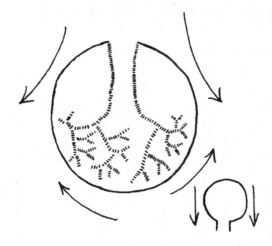

The lung has embarked on this path of development not in order ultimately to create its own air, but to enable it eventually to become the carrier of the air from outside. Through this process, the lung has evolved from being an active air gland in fish into a completely passive organ. The active in-breathing is restrained to allow air to stream in from outside. And to expel the air a 'push' has to come from the direction of the kidneys. Only if we imagine the lung as a completely passive system – it just rests, so to speak – depending on the urogenital system to initiate its activity, only then can we see how the regulation of the intake and release of air is possible.

If we then trace the development of the lung, how the lung is expressed in its many different forms throughout the animal kingdom, and examine this without projecting prejudiced theories of evolution onto the facts, we will, I would propose, find something that is of great importance.

I will give you another example. The lungs of birds – the 'fish of the air' to use an expression from Dr Kolisko – show something that can help us understand what the lung, in its essential nature and gesture, is actually aiming at.[3] The lungs of birds, unlike human lungs (as in the left-hand figure), are not enclosed within the left and right side of the thoracic cavity, but consist of many sacs which extend and grow into the long bones of the birds (right-hand figure). There they replace the bone marrow, where otherwise blood would continually be produced.

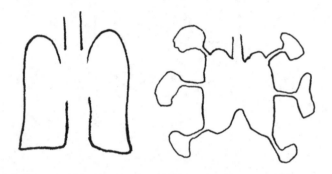

In a bird a certain part of the bone is filled with an air bag. Again we meet the equivalent of the air bladder of fish, but here we meet it more directly. We meet it in a way that it is connected with the particular structure of the species. In fish the ossicles, which connect the air bladder to the organ of balance, show a tendency similar to that of the air bags of birds that do not produce their own air, but fill themselves with outside air. This enables birds to fly and balance in the air.

Connected with this is something that I consider even more important. Around the air bags there is bone marrow, the medulla. This bone marrow is surrounded by blood capillaries corresponding to the relationship in the lungs between the capillaries and the alveoli (figure a). In the bird, however, the surface differs from that of the lung. The millionfold surface area in the lung corresponds to the single, double or tenfold area in the bird.

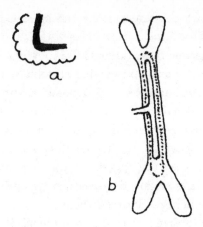

If we regard this as a gesture, what does it imply? Expressed as a kind of inner attitude, the lung organ, which is intimately connected with the whole spatial configuration of the earth, reveals the tendency to relate itself to the nature of the blood. When we study the lung, we find that it has a persistent tendency to relate itself as intimately as possible to the blood. The lung grows as close as possible towards the blood, inclining, as it were, towards the blood.

This is a very intimate gesture. It is a gesture that is often expressed in sculpture, a similar gesture has also been painted many times. It is a gesture reminiscent of the one we find in the description of the Last Supper. Not that I intend to equate the one attitude to the other, but I wish to describe what is at work within the lung, how intimately it inclines towards the chest of the blood as if in longing. This enables the exchange of oxygen and carbon dioxide in the blood.

Here again you have the lung's tendency to renounce itself. This sacrificial tendency of the lungs makes two things apparent. One is that in consequence the cosmic rhythm of 25 920 is able to come to expression. Each day we take as many breaths as there are years in a Platonic Year.[4] This means that the same rhythm, but in a shortened form, pervades both the human being and the

261

universe. We owe this remarkable correspondence to the sacrificial attitude of the lung.

As for the second point, I would like to refer to the third lecture of the Agriculture Course where Rudolf Steiner addressed the nature of carbon. Here we approach more closely what might be the mineral nature, the earthly expression, of the lung. Here Rudolf Steiner tried to reveal the idea to us that carbon is not what he called 'this black fellow' *(schwarzer Kerl),* which we usually picture when thinking of carbon as we see it in coal or graphite. Carbon is actually the substance that enables the cosmic archetypes to enter into organic structure.

Carbon is a substance that continually yields itself to the cosmic archetypes, to the universal pictures underlying all existence. These initially take hold of matter by way of sulphur, through which they connect to carbon. Carbon then takes them up, forms them, dissolves them, forms them and dissolves them again. Then Rudolf Steiner referred to the blood with these words, 'Blood is a very special fluid' *(Blut ist ein ganz besonderer Saft),* because within the blood the human 'I' works and finds its physical expression.[5] Speaking more precisely, more fundamentally, about the working of the human 'I', however, he said that we must acknowledge the task of carbon within the blood, because it is carbon that guides the spirit into matter.

The universal spirit and the human spirit – the universal spirit and the human 'I' – meet when lung and blood come together. The lung has sacrificed itself. Its activity as an organ has become questionable, but in sacrificing itself, it allows the archetypal images to stream in on the rhythm of 25920. There the spirit of the cosmos and the human 'I' meet. The lung is continually striving to be intimately related to the surface of the blood. It meets in the blood this particular capacity working in carbon and which is the working of the individual personality, the 'I'. With such thoughts we take a definite step forward in our quest for understanding, approaching the nature and essence of the lung more closely in the context of the wider organism.

The meeting of blood and lung is also expressed through another important fact, a fact especially relevant for doctors. The human lung (and I say the human lung because here it is especially obvious), has, so to speak, enshrined the heart organ. The left lung has receded and has left part of itself free to surround the heart. This reveals the same gesture as was described earlier, namely the tendency to reach out towards and intimately relate its growth to the blood. Our arms and hands are permeated by the gesture of the lung: they embrace, engage in work, are creative. Our legs, however, are governed by the heart. But of course arms and legs are mutually infused and interact with each other.

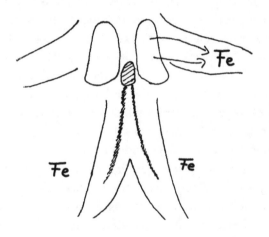

I would have to speak at greater length to characterise the kinds of processes involved here, but a very special stream of iron emanates from the blood and continually counteracts the production of albumen. We will come back to this when we speak about the liver and especially when we speak about the heart itself. Again, this is only a first intimation of what awaits us.

Yesterday we heard how Rudolf Steiner spoke of the organs as being the intuitions of the higher spiritual hierarchies. We will now try to consider the lung in such a way that we ask ourselves:

is it possible to define the intuition of the lung? Some of you will be acquainted with that very significant lecture that Rudolf Steiner gave where he referred to the different nature of the four main organs.[6] He described how human memory is intimately connected with the surface of these organs. He referred to the lung in the following way. The lung takes in, as a memory, thoughts connected with our conception of the world around us, clear-cut forms of ideas, concepts. These clear-cut concepts are taken up through the surface of the lung into the interior of the organ. There they grow into a kind of force or power. After death this power is released. This power grows through the life between death and rebirth, resulting in the configuration of our skull in a subsequent incarnation. Rudolf Steiner portrayed (and this is something that some phrenologists are trying to understand) the surface form of the skull as essentially a reflection of all the concepts and ideas that we assimilated from the outside in a previous life.

But what is the skull? It mirrors the archetypal image of the surface of the earth. The skull is, so to speak, the imprint of the geology of the whole earth. Only when we recognise the truth of this insight can we grasp the full implication of the intimate connection between geology and the lung. This relationship is only fully revealed in the next life, when the inner landscape of concepts is metamorphosed into the structure of the skull. If these formative forces are so strong in this life that they over-power the lung, or if the lung itself in this life is lacking the capacity to contain these forces, then something appears which I tried to describe last night. We stand bewildered in the face of it. We try to avoid confronting it by saying that somebody has become insane. Because, if the forces which are destined to form the skull in the next life already intrude into the soul in this life, the person may develop what we know as obsessive thoughts. In short, paranoid ideas, fixed ideas, emanate from a person in such a condition. This condition reveals the effect of an underlying geological power, but a geology bearing unique personal, earthly ideas and images rather than cosmic, universal archetypes.

I am trying to avoid drawing hard and fast boundaries in these descriptions, and to allow the facts to speak for themselves. In conclusion, I would like to say that the lung occupies a very special position among the four organ systems. The lung normally constitutes the opposite of the forces that are able to stream in through its inner deed of sacrifice. Therefore I have tried to show that the lung as an organ manifests ambivalence. It is a precarious organ with a *transient* nature, so to speak. But, in the metaphor of Goethe's Fairy Tale, we can say that when the call goes out, when the time has come and the Green Snake whispers into the ear of the Old Man, then the time of the Mixed King, the composite, rather awkward figure that I am now connecting with the lung, will have come to an end. Although the lung is destined eventually to collapse, like the Mixed King, we must remember that the Mixed King is not only a ridiculous figure. He has played the most important part in his time which extends into our own. Through cultivating such an understanding of the lung, we will be able to recognise the signs of the lung, which reveal the signs of the times, indicating that the time for change has come. During the last fifteen years a dreadful disease, which until recently was one of the rarest, has become an epidemic all over the civilized world.

Cancer of the bronchial tree has become an epidemic, especially among men, but also among women. There is no doubt that this epidemic is intimately connected with smoking. People are free to evade this issue but in reality it is inescapable. I do not have the impression that it is directly due to the influence of tobacco or nicotine, but that it is rather the other way round. Smoking undermines the upright position of the Fourth King. Smoking (I am staying with the picture) destroys the veins of gold and silver, which originally held the Fourth King in his upright position. As a result of smoking, the ability of the lung organ to adapt to the surrounding nature and geology is completely undermined. Any doctor or farmer who smokes will not be able to sense the geology of the surroundings, because smoking impairs this subtle gift. As a result, the uppermost sphere, the sphere of life of which we spoke last night, is displaced from its rightful cosmic sphere.

Rudolf Steiner described this as a sphere that has to be restrained continually, otherwise, all over the earth, cancerous growths would appear. They will come about if the inner function of the lung fails. These two facts belong together. The powers of life stream in and the cancerous growths come about as a result.

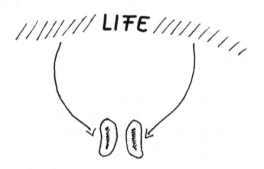

We should become aware that the lung is related to the sphere of life, and that the reign of the Fourth King, which has lasted for a few thousand years, is starting to come to an end.

This is a kind of preliminary introduction to the organ system of the lung. We will refer back to it when speaking about the other three systems.

In answer to a question about breathing through the lungs Karl König gave the following reply.

Rudolf Steiner indicated that the concepts which we have of the world around us, the ordinary concepts that we acquire during our life between birth and death – which have nothing to do with cosmic ideas, but which are the hard and rigid imprints of the surrounding world – are especially connected with the lungs. Furthermore, he referred to the fact that the surface of our lung is an organ bearing the memory of abstract ideas, abstract not in a cosmic but in the concrete, intellectual sense. These spectral ideas have lost their imaginative content.

The lung is therefore related to another phenomenon. You often come across fanaticism, people who are unable to restrain themselves from talking continuously about the same thing. Whenever and wherever you meet this phenomenon, these people continuously bang on about certain things that they are trying to impress upon you. This has to do with the lung. Suppose the lung is not functioning properly. Suppose it does not have the right relation to the rhythm of 25 920, but is trying to become smaller and thereby more effective as a lung. Then it imprints a certain degree of fanaticism. If you start to speak to such people about biodynamics for instance, they will immediately begin to speak about their own particular pet subject, maybe the threefold social order, or something like that.

Each of the organs bears within it the potential for such aberrations. For instance, when speaking to a person influenced by the liver, you may find that you have time to take a walk in the gap between two words, and when you return the next word will follow. This feature has to do with the liver.

I will now mention something else, which gives an entirely new picture of the lung, and yet can also gradually be integrated into what I have tried to unfold this morning. Rudolf Steiner suggested that if you study people suffering from diseases of the lung (and, I would add, especially those who are suffering from tuberculosis), you will notice that they develop very peculiar ideas. There is a famous novel by the German author Thomas Mann, called in English *The Magic Mountain*, which is set in a sanatorium. With great artistic skill, Mann shows how people create a kind of magic world around them. They no longer live in reality. They live in a dream world, which leads progressively to a kind of religious mania.

Now, you can't exactly describe this as the last stage of the geology of the lung, but you can see that it is another manifestation of the intuition of the beings who create the lung. The intimate connection of the lung to the sphere of the planet Venus, which actually implies the sphere of Mercury, becomes evident. In the life between death and rebirth this is the sphere where we receive our religious ideas. You will notice how many things we have to bring together if we want to start to walk in the landscape of the lung. I am convinced that it is the surrounding countryside, the geology of the area where people live, which contributes to the prevalent high incidence of tuberculosis. The fact that certain people live in a dream state is to be attributed to certain geological features.

When I am in Ireland, I am permanently under the impression that there is an enormous power of copper at work. I don't find any iron, however. It may be in the soil, but I am not aware of it. The intense experience one can sometimes have when inhaling an atmosphere filled with the power of iron is simply not there. I would say that here is the egg from which the tuberculosis chicken was hatched: to my mind, it is related to the lack of iron. I believe it is the lack of those substances that have to do with the lung, such as carbon and iron activity. This is my impression, although I have no proof. It is merely a kind of intuition. The first time I was in Ireland and we were travelling by car, I can only say that I was continually aware of a lack of iron. It was simply lacking.

These two, iron and copper, are always in equilibrium with each other. If, for instance, you are investigating blood in which the iron level is reduced, you will inevitably find that the copper level is raised. These two are like a pair of scales. Not only are the planets Venus and Mars opposite to each other in character, but throughout the whole of nature you will always find that they balance each other out. As soon as iron recedes, copper moves in. Iron has to permanently defend itself against the pressure of copper. You can easily understand this when you see it in the following way: copper (and this, of course, is a very subtle process) is related to the process of sprouting – everything that is green is connected with the copper process; whereas iron leads the process of inhalation into every corner of organic life. The plants need an environment of iron.

Both animals and humans need iron as an element within them. It is not a trace element. It is the only metal which is present in substantial form. So I have to describe this iron radiation in connection with the lung, because it forms part of the inhaling process. Iron always (I believe without exception) comes to permeate any growing substance through the process of inhaling. This means that iron is always initiating breakdown processes, whereas copper is essential for all growth processes. This becomes particularly obvious in the study of blood in babies and children in general. It is actually possible to regulate organic functions in children according to their constitution, by means of homoeopathic doses of copper and iron, thereby maintaining a balance. This has been proved scientifically.

We know today that copper plays at least as big a part in blood metabolism as iron. I have the impression that in general terms both tuberculosis and cancer has to do with light. However, tuberculosis of the lung and bronchial cancer are diseases of a special type in that both tuberculosis and cancer can affect any organ of the body. I have the impression that in the nineteenth century, especially during the latter half, under the conditions of the Industrial Revolution, which included child labour, the typical disease was tuberculosis. Nowadays, tuberculosis is decreasing, while cancer is increasing at a similar rate. However, tuberculosis is a general and lung cancer is a particular disease. Lung cancer, or more precisely, bronchial cancer, is a very particular disease, which really has to do with the overpowering forces of the life ether within us. The lung should actually continually be constraining the activity of the life ether.

In his lecture to doctors, when speaking about the sphere of life in connection with the lung, Rudolf Steiner made a very special remark. He said that these overpowering forces must be continually hemmed in, and what must be hemmed in is the power of Mercury. The lung must have the strength to contain the power of Mercury within itself. As soon as the lung is diminished in its power and structure, caused particularly by the inhalation of nicotine and tobacco, these forces break through instead of being contained.

One more point. Mercury is usually associated with the metal mercury. It occupies an unusual position because it is the only metal which remains liquid. I have no proof, but I can only say that I have no doubt that although we are referring to the metal mercury and the power of the metal mercury, we are actually dealing here with the sphere of Venus. It is from this sphere that religious mania originates. When we come to speak about the kidneys we shall have to go into the process of transformation, which took place between Mercury and Venus, when the lung moved from below upwards, just as the kidneys moved from above downwards. Therefore, we have to emphasise once again that in so many respects the lung is a rather ambivalent organ.

3 The Spheres Surrounding the Earth

Lecture 3, Friday, October 31, 1958

I have so far referred in a more or less metaphorical way to the four meteorological spheres of the earth in connection with the four meteorological organs in the human body. In the second lecture we spoke about the organ of the lung. At the end of our morning talk I mentioned the highest sphere, which Rudolf Steiner called the sphere of life or the sphere of the life ether. Tomorrow I will go one step lower and speak about the liver, where we meet the next sphere, the sphere of the chemical or number ether. Below that, we meet the next sphere, where the light originates – not the light of the sun, but the light that sprouts and grows, as Rudolf Steiner said, as the plants grow here on earth – this is the light ether. Only then do we meet the sphere of warmth, the warmth ether, which in us is connected with the heart.

Especially in times like the present the question arises as to where in the surroundings of the earth we can meet these spheres. Are they actually a physical reality? Investigations have been carried out during the last twenty years concerning the different layers and sheaths of the earth. Although it has not so far proved possible to detect these spheres, are there any possible hints as to where these layers may be found? I believe it is necessary to occupy ourselves, at least briefly, with the structure and morphology of these spheres.

It had already become clear during the 1920s and 30s that the sphere of warmth is more distant than had previously been assumed – at a height of about 45 kilometres (30 miles) above the earth. Below this lie the stratosphere and the atmosphere [troposphere]. Beyond the stratosphere, where a layer of ozone is in the process of developing, the temperature suddenly rises to 30°C (85°F).[1] When an explanation for this was found, it ran contrary to everything that had previously been expected. Scientists discovered that in this sphere the ultraviolet light destroys the oxygen atom. As a result of this destruction, warmth is set free, which permeates this whole layer and sphere.

Even Dr Wachsmuth, who made a serious attempt to describe the order of the different spheres – mentioned by Rudolf Steiner – according to the current understanding of the structure of the earthly globe, does not mention these spheres.[2] So I would now like to say a few words about them.

Science has discovered several distinct layers, which are seen as associated with electrical forces. These layers have been named E1 and E2, and F1 and F2. The interesting thing is that these layers appear and disappear. They appear with the rising sun and disappear with the setting sun. Science at present is still unable to interpret their significance. Since I am only a layman in these matters, please take what I have to say with a pinch of salt, but as far as I am informed, science is unable to explain why these layers exist at all. There is no general distribution of electrical potential of any kind in the surrounding layers. These electrical potentials gather together only at certain altitudes. They can be found roughly speaking at an altitude of about 300 km (200 miles), the next one at about 200 km (125 miles) and then again at about 100 km (60 miles).[3]

I am not certain, but it is quite possible that the boundary areas between these ether spheres create layers where the electrical potentials gather together particularly under the influence of the light of the sun. If you permit me to make this very rough estimate, then you may be able to imagine where these four

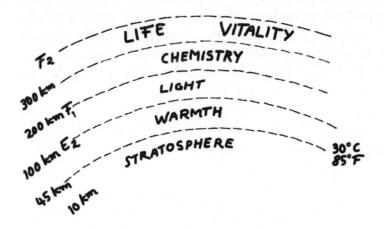

spheres might actually be found. The stratosphere is about 10 km (6 miles) above the earth. Beneath that is everything we experience as the sky and the clouds above us. You must imagine that it is in this very small layer that we have our life and our existence.

All this presupposes that the mantle, the etheric cloak of the earth, would not be worn, torn and tattered. I don't think it is necessary to discuss the tremendous dangers that have arisen during the last ten years through the relatively useless explosion of hydrogen bombs, or the launching of missiles and satellites. All this has gripped our conscience. I hope it has done so very firmly and deeply, because what we are experiencing amounts to the continual, wilful destruction of the atmosphere, the stratosphere, in fact, the whole etheric layering of mother earth. The results are already evident. Further symptoms are bound to make themselves felt, because one cannot expect that in the near future people will develop a better understanding for what they are doing.

These remarks have been offered as a kind of supplement to what we discussed last night. I have felt it necessary to provide a more thorough and more concrete picture of the spheres as a background to our theme.

Now let us return to the four kings in Goethe's Tale. We return to the lung, the heart, the kidney and the liver. We remember carbon, hydrogen, nitrogen and oxygen in relation to earth, water, air and warmth – according to Steiner's medical lecture in March 1920.[4] This is the region we are trying to enter. It is this underground cave where the four kings dwelt and where they can be found. These kings provide a cosmic foundation for our existence. They constitute the intuitions of the spiritual hierarchies which have created physical existence.

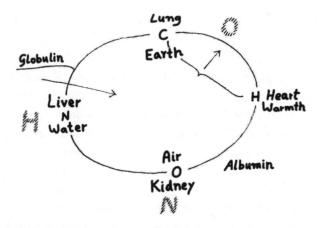

Two and a half years later, in lectures to the members of the Anthroposophical Society in Dornach, and then to a large audience of medical doctors in Stuttgart, Rudolf Steiner spoke again about these four organs, about the elements and about the formation of protein.[5] But on those occasions he spoke in an entirely different way, apparently contradicting all that he had revealed before, connecting oxygen with the heart and lung system. He did not draw a distinction between lung and heart, but spoke about the heart and lung system, which he connected with oxygen, the kidneys still with nitrogen, but the liver with hydrogen; carbon is not mentioned at all.

Now the question arises: who was right? Rudolf Steiner in 1920 or Rudolf Steiner in 1922? How are these two views to be reconciled? Or is it a case of taking either a cosmic or an earthly point of view?

Steiner often pointed out that if one walks around a tree, it will look very different from the other side. But this argument does not appear adequate in this case. If we really follow these lectures, if we really try to understand what Rudolf Steiner was trying to say and what he described, we will gradually discover that these two configurations are entirely different in character. What was Rudolf Steiner in fact describing in 1922? He spoke very movingly and intimately to the members in Dornach, much more movingly than when he was speaking in an emphatic tone to the doctors in Stuttgart. The intimate tone in which he was speaking to the members conveys the impression that he was explaining very significant evolutionary facts.

He spoke in a very moving way about the process of digestion. He described – as he had done many times before – how the process of assimilating food is necessarily connected with the breaking down of all substance, be it mineral, plant or animal. Here he described for the first time, as far as I know, how, when the food has gone through the whole process in mouth, stomach and small intestine, when it is completely broken down, when nothing of its own 'individuality' is left, it assumes, as it were, a condition which he called 'mineral'. He did not say 'physical'. Several times he quite explicitly uses the word 'mineral'. It is now 'mineralised substance,' and as mineral substance it penetrates the walls of the intestines. On the other side it reappears in the lymph vessels – in the lacteals surrounding the intestines. Later on I will refer to the cosmic nutrition stream, about which we must become clear in connection with this very special lecture. Rudolf Steiner went on to describe, in very similar terms, what is known through scientific research: namely that within the lymphatic vessels, this mineral nutrient streams up into the region of the rhythmical organisation, into the region of lung and heart. As yet it remains entirely mineral, however; it is not alive, but it is mere substance.

The lung and heart system then receives this substance. I already tried to encompass the gesture, in an image, this morning, saying that the inner activity of the lung is always inclining with longing towards the blood; that, similarly, in human morphology, the heart is embraced by the lung. These two organs have found each other, so to speak. This is the organisation that now receives mineral substance and permeates it with life. Steiner described this process in the following way: the mineral substance is permeated by the individual ether, by the human etheric body. It is taken up into the etheric body, where it is incorporated through the power of oxygen. The power of oxygen binds the etheric forces to physical existence, and this takes place in the region of heart/lung.

The result, however, is still merely living substance. It is by no means yet *sentient* substance. (Here I am using the terminology that Rudolf Steiner used in the introductory chapters of the medical book, *Extending Medical Practice,* that he later wrote together with Ita Wegman.) In the heart/lung region, the mineral substance becomes living substance. Now, however, the food has to be brought into the sentient condition, into what is called the astral body. This only happens through the forces which stream from the region of the kidneys.

From the kidneys, the astral forces penetrate the living substance, which then takes a further step in the direction of becoming humanised. Here, Steiner indicated that it is the element of nitrogen which enables the food that so far has only been enlivened, to become sentient substance. It becomes part of our astral nature. It is still not completely individualised. It will only become completely human if our own individuality can permeate it and make it its own, through the I-organisation.

This happens, according to these lectures by Steiner, through the forces of hydrogen, not now from the region of the heart, but entirely from the region of the liver and the gall bladder. Rudolf

Steiner did not speak here only of the liver. He spoke of the combined system of liver and gall bladder. He clearly described this liver and gall bladder system as a system that is intimately connected to the 'I' itself. He even said that in evolution you will find that the liver and gall bladder are properly developed only where the higher animals are approaching the possibility of receiving into themselves the 'I'. When this has been achieved, when the forces of hydrogen bind the 'I' to substance, and the substance has been taken up into the whole of our existence, including our I-organisation, only then does the food finally become individualised: Nutrition has then fulfilled its task.

This is a very powerful picture, corresponding to what is indeed a very powerful process that we are following here. However, one question remains to be answered: Where does the cosmic nutrition stream fit in? At this point, Rudolf Steiner was speaking about earthly nutrition, following this earthly nutrition stream through our intestines into the entire system of our bodily existence – etheric, astral and 'I'. The question remains as to how the cosmic nutrition stream is connected to the earthly process. Has it been left out entirely? Rudolf Steiner pointed to the fact that only certain parts of our forebrain take up all that we receive through the earthly nutrition stream. All other substances making up our body are, he said, the result of the cosmic nutrition stream, which streams into our existence by way of the sense organs.[6]

It is of the greatest importance that we do not ignore such descriptions, that we do not speak about earthly nutrition on one occasion and on another about cosmic nutrition. If we do not consider both types of nutrition in their mutual relationship, if we do not at least attempt some kind of synthesis of what Rudolf Steiner said, we restrict our possibilities of deeper understanding.

Speaking now only on the basis of my personal understanding, I do not have the impression that beyond the intestinal wall this mineralised substance to which Rudolf Steiner referred remains confined to the earthly nutrition stream. We know that the mineral substance enters into these vast realms of lymph, into which cosmic nutrition also streams. There the mineralised, broken-down substance coming from earthly nutrition enters and permeates the extensive system of lacteals in the areas surrounding the intestines, especially the small intestine.[7] There it meets, mixes and unites with the substances of the cosmic nutrition stream. This happens because humans are only partly cosmic beings, and do not easily digest the cosmic nutrition stream, just as we would not be able to endure the earthly nutrition stream unless its substance were first broken down.

In the cosmic nutrition stream, however, there is no actual substance that needs to be broken down. The cosmic nutrition stream, composed of etheric forces, enters our organism through our whole etheric organisation. It rains down and settles in the lymphatic system as physical, mineral substance. These two streams then unite and together they are taken up and individualised. Out of them we make, with the help of oxygen, nitrogen, hydrogen and the four organs, the individualised nutritional substance. This is the first step.

Now we can see how the four kings are placed within the physical realm of our bodily nature. Surrounding them we may picture the spheres of the earth – of the existing layers of the earthly sheaths. In a corresponding way, they are present within us, where they have remained static. They are like pillars, and surrounding them, continually in the ether realm, there is this atmosphere of primeval albumen, which once surrounded our globe. This primeval atmosphere of albumen now exists as an individualised drop within us. It is, as it were, in a process of continuous becoming. Into this, however, enters something entirely different, namely the whole earthly nutritional stream that I have just described. According to Rudolf Steiner, this is not a static stream, but a stream of coming into being and dissolving.

These four organs, in the form in which they represent the four kings, have nothing to do with binding the etheric, the astral and the 'I' to the physical. They are not concerned with the individualisation of the nutrition stream. As in a vast cell, they create protein and, through that creation, warmth, air, fluid and earth – the four elements – arise. Where physical and etheric are united, like two clasped hands, the continuous creation of protein is carried on in these four elements.

During the last twenty years, scientists have discovered a tremendous amount of information about protein, and especially about the proteins contained in our blood plasma. Though unable to account for it, they have been compelled to distinguish between two kinds of proteins – the albumins and the globulins. Today we know that the amounts of albumen and globulin vary considerably in different people, with different diseases, and at different ages.

I will give you one example. The globulins are subdivided into alpha, beta, gamma and so on. I believe that in infancy and early childhood the amount of albumins is higher than the amount of globulin. The same holds good for the growing child, where the albumins are between 60 and 70% higher. However, it has been discovered, for instance, that in children with Down syndrome the amount of globulins in the blood plasma is higher than in other people. The amount of globulin in the embryo is also particularly high.

Science has not yet discovered the exact composition of albumins, except for one particular part of the structure (a discovery for which the Nobel Prize was awarded).[8] But I would consider that the globulins are what one might call the macrocosmic protein, whereas the albumins are much more microcosmic. So perhaps one may now begin to understand how the globulins continually arrive in this sphere of existence of the four kings. They might more or less be called the cosmic protein. The albumins, however, derive from both the cosmic and the earthly nutrition streams. These streams mix in the blood plasma, in the blood serum. There they determine our existence – or we determine theirs – however you like to express it. But we must learn to distinguish these two processes.

A closer look at the simple diagram (p. 274) will give a reliable key to understanding this process very clearly. Earth and warmth signify the whole spectrum in the manifestation of the four elements. (I am not referring to the chemical elements, but to earth, air, water and fire in the sense in which Hippocrates and Paracelsus spoke about them.) Between earth and warmth – between lung and heart – there streams oxygen. Oxygen makes itself at home in the whole ether body, becoming part of the mineralised nutrition and raising it up into vitalised substance.

Then we come to the element of air, where the astral body lives. Here nitrogen, the power that binds astrality into the physical substance, arises and unfolds. This is the second step.

With the third step the action moves up into the sphere of the liver and the gall bladder. There it meets hydrogen and leads all this into the 'I'.

Tomorrow we will speak more about the middle system. We will start with the question of nitrogen, hydrogen and the blood. These considerations presuppose an understanding of albumins and globulins as two kinds of protein, one being more individual (not earthly but human, and the other more cosmic). We cannot simply equate hydrogen with the 'I' or oxygen with the etheric body. In the first formula which Rudolf Steiner gave about the protein-formation process, he confines himself to the sphere of the elements, because here the picture of cosmic protein is being built up through the image of the elements as they were understood in antiquity, although he now places them into the context of medical science. This is to be seen as a static process, the other as a dynamic one. The static process corresponds to the formation of cosmic protein and the more dynamic one to the formation of human protein. When understood in this way, these two processes no longer appear as mutual contradictions, but reveal the possibility of interpreting these matters in a true light.

4 The Liver

Lecture 4, Saturday, November 1, 1958

As an echo to our discussion of the lung, I would like to read the passage from *The Portal of Initiation*, Rudolf Steiner's first Mystery Drama, which George Adams mentioned yesterday. He made me aware of words that I had completely forgotten. Towards the end of the fifth scene, which takes place in the temple, Retardus, who is the figure corresponding to the Fourth (or Mixed) King, speaks to the other three kings:

> If they unite with you,
> what will become of me?
> My deeds will then prove fruitless
> For pupils of the spirit path.
>
> BENEDICTUS: You will transform to other life
>   for you have done your work.
> THEODOSIUS: You will live on in sacrifice
>   If you will sacrifice yourself.
> ROMANUS: You will bear fruit in human deeds,
>   If I can cultivate the fruit.[1]

One could hardly find a more wonderful justification for what I have tried to express about the lung. It happens repeatedly that when we join our efforts to find answers to our questions, words are found that reinforce what we have come to. If some of you are planning a more detailed study of these four kings, please don't forget what I have just read to you. Our thanks go to Mr Adams for making us aware of this connection.

Before embarking on our study of the liver – another organ corresponding to one of the four kings in the underground temple – I would like to point to a more imaginative way of envisioning the work of the four main protein-building organs.

Let us now turn to the third lecture of Steiner's Agricultural Curse, which probably constitutes the centre of the entire course. With great and ever renewed effort Rudolf Steiner was trying to convey to us something about the four main substances, the four main chemical elements that constitute the substance known as albumen or protein. In order to bring them closer to our understanding, he discusses them from many different aspects. Time and again we need to study anew his very complicated sentences and expressions; within them the foundation for our understanding of all organic life is to be found. We are being invited to observe, from our human point of view, the workings of carbon, hydrogen, nitrogen, and oxygen.

Both visual and conceptual help in this task will be gained if we take up as a comparative study the lectures given by Rudolf Steiner in 1921, in which he called upon the artist in each of us and attempted to convey a certain understanding of colours.[2] He named four so-called image colours, green, black, white and peach-blossom. In describing them, he characterised green as the dead image of life, peach-blossom as the living image of the soul, white as the soul-life image of the spirit, and black as the spiritual image of death.

If you now try to grasp the fact that green is the dead image of life, that it is no longer life itself, but its image, that in it, life has already more or less come to an end, then you can compare this characterisation to a sentence from the third lecture of the Agriculture Course, where Rudolf Steiner, referring to oxygen, said that the oxygen around us must be devitalised, despite the fact that, from birth onwards, oxygen is the carrier, the bearer of life, of ether. Nitrogen carries life into form, which is embodied in carbon. He then said, wherever there is nitrogen, there is astrality. Now you know that this is peach-blossom. It is the living image of the soul. Wherever there is nitrogen, there is astrality. It leads life into the form of carbon, so that, chemically, nitrogen is astral and oxygen is etheric. It would be jumping to conclusions to say that 'nitrogen is astrality.' There is world astrality, and this world astrality leads life into form. This relates to peach-blossom. With this we are actually saying much more than when we say that nitrogen brings astrality to manifestation.

In a similar way hydrogen is white and carbon is black; this means that coal is ultimately black. This is the key to understanding the mystery of carbon. Then you can begin to imagine hydrogen as the spiritual image of the soul. Similarly, you can speak of carbon as related to death, albeit the spiritual image of death.

Carbon
black

Nitrogen   Hydrogen
peach blossom   white

green
Oxygen

I wanted to point to this imagination in the same way as when yesterday morning I pointed to the four kings in their form and being. Now we can refer to the kings and realise that they do not simply equate to physical, etheric, astral and 'I'. By no means. You need to be aware that as soon as activity connects with earth existence, there is always a continuous ebbing and flowing, building up and breaking down, a flowing, dynamic nature.

If we now add colour to this activity and look at the realm of verdant life in the knowledge that it is the dead image of life, we will meet to a certain extent the nature and essence of oxygen. Similarly, if we see peach-blossom, we will meet the nature of nitrogen. So if we now embark on the study of the liver, we enter in a cloud of peach-blossom, as it were. Then we come close to nitrogen, then we can try to imagine nitrogen, and in nitrogen to discover the living image of the soul. These imaginations are working and weaving in the liver, albeit more or less unconsciously

This may serve as a path to what we discussed last night. Not until we have reached a certain understanding of those processes we mentioned will we be able to reach an understanding of the organ-system of the liver. It is no doubt the most complicated system of the four, because it is so all-encompassing. As in no other organ, the greatest secrets are enshrined in the liver. On entering the liver, we may imagine that we are entering the place where the Bronze King of Goethe's Fairy Tale is standing; and where the Bronze King stands, the greatest mystery of earthly existence is concealed. This is the secret of the liver.

Enshrined in the liver is the centre of our will-existence, the centre of our life, the intentionality underlying our action and work, the will power underlying our very existence. These powers are enclosed in the liver, not merely in the physical organ, but in the etheric realm, in the realm of the elements. Here nitrogen has its place.

Last night we spoke of how hydrogen has its existence in relation to the human 'I', in so far as the stream of nutrition is inspirited by its *organ*. In this drawing, I am trying to make this visible. Above we have carbon, then here is the heart and hydrogen, and finally the kidneys and oxygen. Yesterday we referred to this as the static cosmic sphere of the formation of protein. In the primeval phase of earth evolution the prototype of this protein sphere was the sheath of the earth, where breathing and nutrition were still united, not physically, but only in the realm of the

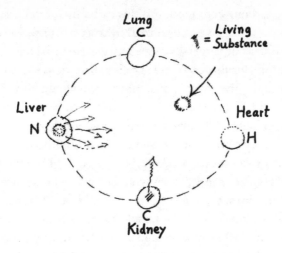

ether permeating the physical structure, thereby precipitating out the four elements of fire and air, water and earth.

Then we have another process, a dynamic process, which leads the mineralised food on the path to becoming the substance of the human being. It is here that oxygen streams in, turning the black mineral food substance into living substance. It is turned green. Then with the help of nitrogen in the region of the kidneys, this greening, living substance is made into sentient substance, and thereby becomes incorporated sentient existence. Finally, with the help of hydrogen, it becomes truly a part of us. It becomes 'I'.

Earlier I described how both the earthly and the cosmic nutrition streams become woven together in us, the one more in the form of albumins, and the other more in the form of globulins. On the one hand is the more static etheric sphere, guarded by the four kings, and on the other hand, a kind of dynamic, continuous process of the shaping of digested food, humanised through oxygen, nitrogen and hydrogen.

Carbon does not feature here at all, because the mineralised food, in the way in which it is broken down in our intestines, is itself the carbon, so to speak. To this carbonised food, oxygen is introduced, nitrogen is introduced, hydrogen is introduced, and so it becomes our very own substance. We can build our body by means of it. But this can happen only when the static sphere of the four kings, the creators of albumin, provide the foundation.

So on the living stage of this cosmic protein creation, the dynamic creation of human protein is continually taking place. I have already pointed out how mineralised food becomes living food: the broken-down food, beyond the wall of the intestines, in the lymphatic lacteals, mixes with the rain of the cosmic nutrition stream; from there it streams upwards from this area.

There is a particular large lymph vessel that carries this food upwards from below into the upper circulation, very close to the region of heart. Now the enlivening process begins. The liver is

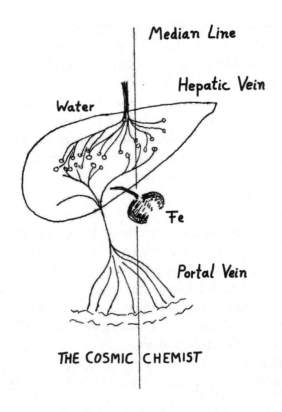

286

a huge organ. It is virtually the largest organ in the body. From the right hand side of the abdomen, it reaches over into the left side. This would be roughly the median line.

Science generally conveys the picture that everything that is digested is taken up directly either into the portal capillaries, joining the portal vein, whereby the digested food is carried into the liver, or that it is taken up directly into the lacteals of the lymphatic system, from where it flows directly into the systemic venous circulation near the heart. Obvious as this simplified interpretation would appear to be from the standpoint of standard physiology, it does not fully satisfy me on the basis of everything I have learned through Rudolf Steiner.[3] My difficulty with it is that it assumes a transfer of substances from the intestinal tract to the blood or to the lacteals, while ignoring the fact that it is first gathered together on the other side of the intestinal wall within the extra cellular spaces that are filled with tissue fluid. This intermediate transition stage has thereby been missed out, on the assumption that it is of no special significance; yet it is just in this transition that I suspect the forces of cosmic nutrition play their role.[4]

The liver as such can be understood only if it is seen as an organ that extends between two venous circulations. It has very little connection with the arterial circulation. This should become a guiding principle for doctors considering liver disease, because the supply of oxygen to the liver always tends to be slightly deficient. If this were not the case, the liver would not be able to function as it does. Yet for all the questions and problems surrounding liver pathology, this lack of oxygen is a decisive factor when considering the nature of the activity of the liver.

You see how this portal vein extends its sinusoidal branches throughout the liver like a tree, and how eventually this blood flows into the hepatic vein. Out of minute twigs and tributaries the substantial stem of the hepatic vein develops, joining the inferior vena cava, which then penetrates the diaphragm, and finally enters the heart.

The crowns of the two huge trees link the tree of the portal vein and the tree of the hepatic vein; the leaves between these two trees link the two circulations together, so to speak. The entire activity of the liver takes place in the sphere of these leaves, and just as every plant leaf has two sides, an upper one and a lower one, so – still using the same image – each liver leaf has the equivalent of an upper and a lower side: the lower one belongs to the hepatic side; the upper one belongs to the portal side. The orientation is inverted, so to speak. I would like to say the moon of the portal vein, not the sun shines on the upper side, although it corresponds to the lower leaves of the liver, while the lower side belonging to the hepatic vein corresponds to the light side. The orientation is reversed.

If you imagine that every minute about two litres of blood flows through the liver, you will understand what Paracelsus meant when he described the liver in his *Tractatus*.[5] His words could be freely rendered by saying: 'If these Galenic idiots' – he was referring to his contemporary colleagues – 'knew how much water flows through and is created in our own organism – which is as if Moses were continually tapping with his rod on the liver and thereby opening a continuously flowing spring – they would also be able to consider the right remedies.' This flowing, continuous stream of fluid, which pours through the liver, can be regarded as acting in conjunction with nitrogen, because the power and essence of nitrogen is condensed in the liver. Nitrogen, which in the cosmos is dispersed, is concentrated in the liver. This picture offers an appropriate starting point for a discussion of the manifold metabolic processes in the liver.

Almost everything that takes place within the realm of metabolism is carried out by the liver. Through its active chemistry, for instance, the liver maintains the level of blood sugar, of glycogen. I can't go into details and describe to you what this means; suffice it to say that if this level were not maintained, our 'I' would not be able to maintain itself within the blood. If the blood sugar level rises too high or falls too low, our 'I' leaves its physical abode, the blood, and consciousness is affected in two ways. Either we sink into the oblivion of our own body, or we are enveloped in a realm beyond physical existence.

These two different kinds of unconsciousness arise when blood sugar levels are not maintained within their healthy physiological range. The work of maintaining equilibrium is done by the liver. The leaves, or more precisely, the liver cells, continually store the glycogen that they extract from the circulating blood, or they return it to the circulating blood as required in the form of glucose. We must imagine that the leaves of the liver are continually monitoring the chemical composition of the blood serum. This is like an active listening, because if there is too little in the blood, more is supplied, and if there is too much, sugar is taken out and stored in the liver as glycogen. The liver needs to maintain a continuous awareness of the flowing bloodstream.

This applies not only to the level of blood sugar. Urea metabolism, which stands in the background of sugar metabolism, has to do with nitrogen. Urea is not only maintained, it is actually created almost exclusively in the liver. Urea is continually being created in order to prevent an overload of the toxic nitrogenous by-products of protein metabolism. The liver also plays a central role in the catabolism of haemoglobin, a specific protein that forms the inner scaffold of red blood cells. Bilirubin, a component of bile, is a by-product of this breakdown process. In the bone marrow new haemoglobin can then be generated. At the same time, the iron that has been extracted from the haemoglobin molecules is retained within the body, being either stored in the liver or released into the blood. If you imagine this complex of metabolic processes, you will appreciate the key position occupied by the liver with respect to maintaining the entire structure of the blood.

So far the liver has only been described as a kind of servant within the metabolism. Through an activity of inner listening, it serves the chemical needs of the organism, but when considering its role in the formation of bile, the liver takes up its own more assertive position as an exocrine gland in its own right. Imagine for a moment how bees assert themselves when they inject poison; in a similar way liver cells, which may also be pictured as bees, swarming between the two trees of the portal and hepatic veins, create bile. Alongside each liver cell the minute bile capillaries are situated. You can imagine millions of them relieving the liver of a certain congestion, and excreting the bile via the gall bladder and bile ducts into the duodenum. Once the bile has entered the duodenum, it immediately assumes a key role in the breakdown of fats taken in by way of nourishment. In this respect, too, the liver holds overall responsibility.

When creating bile and functioning as a gland within its own realm, the liver assumes its position as an organ of will. The production of bile contains the secret that is connected with this very power. It also is the place where iron is working as a cosmic force, and where the power of the planet Mars is working. When we look around us and when we see the glorious colourings of the trees in autumn, we should remember that the same process, *only in reverse,* is continually taking place within the liver organ. This is evident even in the colouring, because bile, coming from 'liver bees' or 'liver trees', is reddish brown. Only gradually, as it flows out of the organ through the bile duct and is then concentrated in the gall bladder, does it turn green. Here we see a process that is the reverse of what we see outside in the plant world, which start as green and end as reddish-brown.

There are many other matters that ought to be described in this connection. One of these, which I would like to point out to you now, I had already mentioned when I spoke to you in Clent about the sheaths of the biodynamic preparations.[6] I pointed out that the liver is an organ that is inserted into the twenty-four hour time rhythm, not of the human 'I', but of the rotation of the earth. You can also read about this in Dr Wachsmuth's book, *The Etheric Formative Forces.* He says that bile and sugar – the production of bile and glycogen – are two processes that do not occur at the same time, but alternate rhythmically throughout the day. They are distributed in such a way that bile production takes place as a day activity and sugar production as a night activity. Bile production begins in the early morning when the sun is rising, whereas glycogen production is greatest at night, when the sun is shining *through* the earth.[7]

The power of the midnight sun is contained in the glycogen. The power of the midday sun is in the bile. This alteration has been proven, because when people travel from Europe to America, the liver rhythm readjusts according to the new region. The liver is dependent on its position with respect to the earth's rotation in relation to the sun. Now you can imagine why Rudolf Steiner called it a meteorological organ. For when the entire water content of the surroundings changes – which is of course also dependent on light and darkness – the liver also changes.

Nowadays the liver is an organ that is under severe attack from the effects of modern civilisation. The liver is an organ which during the last ten years has started to suffer increasingly under the impact of the modern way of life. What I am going to say now is but a repetition of what physicians from both America and Germany have recently been bringing to our attention.

Today an illness that was relatively unknown twenty or thirty years ago is beginning to reach epidemic proportions. A doctor might have seen a case two or three times a year, but now what is called 'epidemic' jaundice, a jaundice induced by a virus, is encountered more frequently.[8] This is a kind of jaundice that directly and immediately attacks liver cells. It causes the oxygen level of the liver to fall below the level required for normal liver function. You will appreciate what I mean when I say that the lifeblood of our existence is drained away by this illness.

People who have suffered from jaundice and have not received appropriate treatment have considerable difficulty in recovering their initiative, their inner strength of will, their capacity for presence of mind or their ability actively to confront the requirements of earthly existence. Jaundice resembles poliomyelitis in some respects, and the virus is probably similar.[9]

Jaundice also penetrates to the centre of our existence, into the region where our volition is at the disposal of our own 'I', our individuality, our I am.

Increasingly this form of jaundice is spreading. It is probably able to develop because the quality of our food is continually falling and eventually becomes so mineralised that the living powers of oxygenation, on which the liver depends, are not able to reach it.[10] We should bear this in mind, because it refers to what Rudolf pointed to in the lectures of October 1922.[11] He said that our modern consciousness depends upon proper liver function.

Lastly, I would like to say something about the divine intuition out of which the liver is created. In the same way that the surface of the lung reflects the memories of abstract thoughts, the ordinary ideas and concepts of the world around us, so the surface of the liver is especially connected with images warmed through with sentiment, with thoughts enlivened by comfortable feelings. When our physical body is laid down at the portal of death, when our ether body unites with the ether of the whole cosmos and when our astrality expands into the far distances, then what is stored in the liver as heart-filled, heart-warmed thought is taken up and goes through the metamorphosis of the existence between death and rebirth. On returning, it does not become the skull formation as is the case with the abstract thoughts that were connected with the lung of the previous life, but creates the structure of our brain in the next life.

Rudolf Steiner described that our way of thinking depends on the disposition of the brain (not the form of the brain, but the disposition of the brain that is brought about by the memory of the feeling-imbued thoughts of the previous life).[12] Whether we are penetrating thinkers, who follow a thought through to the end, or whether our thoughts are flowing and floating around all over the place, just touching a bit here and there, depends on the disposition of the brain, which is created by what has previously lived in us. If, however, these powers are already pressed out in this life, if the liver is not strong enough to contain them, or if they are too strong to be held by the liver – then our waking consciousness is subsumed by visions and hallucinations of all kinds, rising up into consciousness. Visionaries and mystics are all in some way dependent on those cosmic intuitions which once built the liver and now stream out in a humanised way, in an individualised, personal way.

Such images can sometimes be very beautiful. On the other hand, if the liver becomes congested, so that the concentration of the bile thickens, then human will-power falls to a low ebb. We become not only mentally enfeebled, but also stubborn. The capacity to make decisions is lost; we confront the world without being able to decide what action to take, where to go or how to act.

You see, all these considerations belong to the sphere of the liver, because the liver contains water; with the water, chemical activity is brought down from the sphere surrounding the earth. The liver contains nitrogen, which is the peach-blossom, the carrier of astrality; there, astrality is introduced into the element of water. In the centre there is hydrogen, as the expression of the individual 'I', where the individual will resides. Rising upward from below, and sinking downwards from above into our individual existence, the liver acts and works.

I fully appreciate that what I have tried to describe in this lecture is nothing but an incomplete, very modest and extremely inadequate attempt to portray the vastness and magnitude of this organ, the organ of the Bronze King, the one who says, 'The sword into the left hand and the right hand free.' That is the liver.

Discussion

A question was asked about sunlight and moonlight on the 'leaves' of the surface of the liver.

Karl König: This was only intended as an imaginative picture, and is not referring to the actual moonlight, but is meant to indicate that the upper part of the liver cells corresponds to the lower part of the leaves of the plants outside. What in the plant turns towards the light, in the liver turns the other way round. What in the plant is turned towards the ground, in the liver is turned upwards. This is the orientation. But again, it should not be imagined that each liver cell has exactly the same two surfaces as the leaves of plants. What I mean is that the two functions of each liver cell – the building up of glycogen sugar on the one hand and the formation of bile on the other – correspond to the upper and the lower sides of the leaf in plants. This is connected to the rising and setting sun and to the twenty-four hour rhythm of the rotation of the earth around its axis, and not to our own internal rhythm, the twenty-four hour rhythm of the 'I'. Therefore the one side of the liver is turned towards the sun and bile is produced; the other side is turned towards the moon, towards the night, and sugar is produced. These are the two sides of the liver cell, which correspond to the two sides of the leaves, not so much in form but in function.

Question: Is the liver function different in winter and in summer?
Karl König: I am convinced that there is a very marked difference in liver function during winter and summer, only we have as yet no proof, nor am I aware of any direct indications from Rudolf Steiner about a difference in function. On the other hand we have another indication in one of his lectures to workmen, to the effect that human physiology is different in the cooler and

in the equatorial regions.[13] The relation between lung and liver is different in the polar region and in the region of the equator; the lungs are relatively larger in the polar region, while the liver is much stronger and bigger in the equatorial region.

As soon as we grasp this, we can see how the difference between Eskimos or Inuit and Negroes is determined by this relationship. Modern science does not see it like that, but it is possible to approach differences between the constitution of Inuit and the constitution of people who have grown up in equatorial regions from a phenomenological perspective. It is evident that in the latter the metabolic system – the chemistry – is much more robust, much more in the foreground, virtually overpowers everything else. In Inuit it is more the contemplative life, the reflective life, which predominates, as the lung is much more strongly developed. These are, of course, the fundamentals of what Rudolf Steiner, following Hippocrates, called 'geographic medicine', and which he encouraged us to develop.[14] Needless to say, it will need a great deal of research, and the involvement of thousands of doctors and scientists will be required, if this approach is to be properly grounded.

There is no doubt, however, that every region has its own particular effect on human existence. You only need to consider how language and gestures are influenced by the particular region. And all this, of course, goes much deeper. If you are greeted, for example, with the characteristic gesture of a person from the north-east of Scotland, you will know where he hails from, even if you meet him in South Africa. You will never see a Yorkshire man greet you in quite the same manner, and a Londoner will do it differently again. Everything is connected with the region. We are far from knowing all the details of how all this comes about.

Question: Do you think that the sugar and the glycogen in our blood are formed by the midnight sun, and the starch and the sugar in the plant leaf by the daytime sun?

Karl König: Exactly! Only do not say in the *blood,* but in the *liver.* Glycogen is formed in the liver and from there it is poured into the blood as sugar and it is then transported to the muscles via the blood. The actual production of glycogen takes place in the liver.

Question: Is it right to think that energy and muscular movement are in some way based on the oxidation of glycogen?

Karl König: As long as you say 'in some way,' I would be able to affirm it. If you were to say 'entirely' the statement would be unjustified. We still do not know enough about how the energy of muscular movement comes about. Even with the most detailed experiments, we have not yet been able to discover the actual metabolism within the striated muscles. Many different substances – glycogen among them – play a significant role, but this is only a part of what really takes place. I can't give you a more detailed account, because it still remains to be discovered.[15]

A question was asked about the chemical ether and the life forces of the liver.

Karl König: It is possible for three-quarters of the liver to be destroyed, and the remaining quarter will then regenerate; the liver mass of the last quarter will enlarge to three, four or five times its original size, compensating for what has been lost. You must imagine the liver as a continually sprouting organ. I think I have mentioned this already. If, for instance, you were to remove the right kidney, the liver would quickly grow into the space previously occupied by the kidney. It is a kind of ever-expanding power and force. You only need to imagine that every minute two litres of blood streams through the liver. Just imagine what this means. It means 120 litres per hour! How much is that per day? Almost three thousand litres [almost 800 US gallons] of blood pass through the liver every day! This means that three thousand litres of blood are listened to, that three thousand litres are continually being changed and worked through. That is work indeed!

George Adams: With regard to geographical medicine: I remember that somewhere Rudolf Steiner, speaking about history and the epochs of civilisation, said that one can get a kind of physiological perception of an area. He said that when one contemplates the ancient Egyptian civilisation one gets a feeling of 'liver'.

Karl König: As far as I remember, it is in lectures that Rudolf Steiner gave in 1914, when he explained the columns of the first Goetheanum. I cannot recall it exactly, but he speaks about Egypt as connected with Jupiter, and therefore with the liver.[16]

George Adams: In connection with legumes, there is a sentence in the Agriculture Course which we have always had difficulty understanding. It is where Rudolf Steiner, speaking of the leguminous plants and their green colour, said something about the winter. Now I, and I am sure other friends in the agricultural movement, would be very grateful if you could throw some light on this.
The following passage was then read.

> ... these plants tend to keep what lives in nitrogen very
> close to the ground – in fact, they carry it into the ground
> – while the other plants develop it higher up. You can
> see how the legumes tend to color their leaves somewhat
> darker green than other plants. You can also notice that
> the actual fruits of these plants are somehow stunted,
> as it were, and that their seeds lose their viability quite
> quickly. These plants, in fact, are organised in such a way
> as to bring to expression what the plant world receives
> from the winter, not from the summer. Therefore it
> could be said: In these plants there is always the tendency
> to wait for winter; they would actually like to wait for
> winter with what they develop. Their growth slows down
> when they find enough of what they really need, enough
> nitrogen in the air, which in their own fashion they are
> able to carry downward.[17]

Karl König: There is actual stunting of the fruit. This I think is the crucial point. From what we have just heard, I get the impression that the legumes very much fit into this picture of the liver. They tend very much more to the side of the bile and therefore lose the sugar aspect to a certain degree. What this aspect is exactly I am not sure, but I will think about it.

George Adams: Morphologically, I have always felt that this particular characteristic can be observed if you look at the fruit-formation process of the leguminous plants. I think there is hardly any other kind of plant in which the leaf form is so pervasive. It is as though the sphere of the flowering and fruiting process had been carried down into the region of leaf formation. The pea pod looks like two leaves joined together, so that the fruiting process appears carried down into the region of the leaf. That I can understand, but what he says about winter and summer I don't understand.

It seems as though through nitrogen – what you called peach-blossom, the peach-blossom colour of the whole region of the flower – the whole universe is working in the coloured world of flowers through the power of nitrogen. All the flower colours actually originate from peach-blossom. Whereas in other flowering plants the nitrogen remains in that realm, so that it only enters the material of the rest of the plant to a delicate degree, in beans and peas it enters into the material substance of the plant to a considerable degree. This is the big difference. I once heard someone – I believe it was at Penmaenmawr – ask Dr Steiner whether it was true that beans were bad. Dr Steiner answered, 'Everything is bad for something.' Then he went on, smiling but quite serious, 'Beans are bad for the faculty of perceiving the secrets of numbers in the universe.' I've never forgotten that reference to the secret of numbers.

Karl König: The secret of numbers, which is Pythagorean, is intimately connected with the chemical forces of our organisation. For there lies the secret of numbers: how substances combine with others in relationships of ones, twos, threes, fours, sevens or tens. In this way one might imagine how the realms of the beans and the secret of numbers are connected.

George Adams: And can we conclude from this that the liver is the chemist?

Karl König: Yes!

George Adams: And that the chemical ether is also the number ether?

Karl König: Yes!

5 The Kidney

Lecture 5, Sunday, November 2, 1958

In this lecture we will enter the sphere of the kidneys. This means that we are today concerned especially with the realm of the Silver King. In the first scene of Goethe's Fairy Tale, when the Old Man with the Lamp appears in the cave of the kings, there is a short conversation between him and the Silver King. The Silver King asks, 'Will my kingdom end?' and the Old Man replies, 'Late or never.' In a way this sentence is a kind of prophecy, but it can also help us to discover how this relates to the very special realm of the kidneys.

We should try with our thinking to penetrate such an organ on a deeper level rather than immediately addressing its physiological and pathological expression. For these organs are the sense organs of higher beings, and as such they bear the destiny, the karma, the *whole evolution* of these beings within them. This means that the kidney has a destiny that we can describe in a similar way to that of the lung and the liver, which we considered earlier.

The kidney has a very special destiny, a destiny very different from that of the other three organ systems. Perhaps in considering these words 'late or never,' we can see that the kidney is embedded fully and totally in the history of mankind. 'Late or never' would imply that the destiny of the Silver King is to be fulfilled only when the destiny of mankind on earth has been redeemed.

We shall now try to visualise the physical form, the morphology, of the kidneys. Underneath the vault of the diaphragm, we see two long strands, the ureters, reaching down from the kidneys and ending in the urinary bladder. This immediately reveals a quite different structure and form to that of the liver, in the first place because we are dealing with two symmetrical organs. There is one liver, but there are two kidneys. If we wish to understand this symmetrical form we have to consider another organ, which is also twofold and relatively symmetrical: the lungs and the bronchial tree. The kidneys are really the living image, albeit the reflected image, of the lungs, and vice versa. The mirror itself is the diaphragm; above the diaphragm the lungs mirror the kidneys and below the diaphragm, the kidneys mirror the lungs.

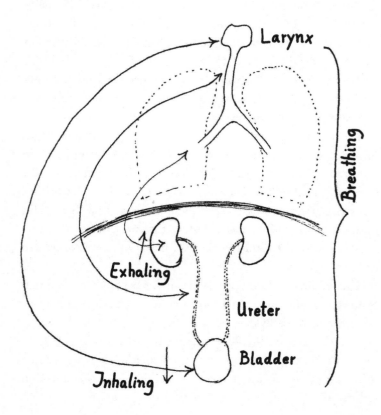

Nevertheless it would be quite wrong merely to state that the kidneys are a mirror image of the lungs, that they mirror each other – the one above, the other below the surface of the diaphragm. We can also understand that not only does the upper side of the kidneys mirror the lower side of the lungs and vice versa, but also that the bladder mirrors the larynx, and the single urethra (through which the urine exits the bladder) mirrors the windpipe or trachea. In this way you will be able to see how living mirror images are to be found within the bodily organisation.

The entirety of what we have just described, rather than merely the one or the other organ, the entire structure of the lung, together with the kidney system, constitutes the organ of breathing. In discussing the lung I described how the bladder pulls and sucks, and how the kidney itself pushes, so that inhaling and exhaling are actively performed. The result of this inhaling and exhaling shows itself in the expansion and contraction of the chest, resulting in the intake and expulsion of air from the lung. But you cannot equate the breathing process simply with the lung. This is where the physical expression of the breathing process is manifest, but the act of breathing, the pull of *inhaling* and the push of *exhaling* resides with the kidney-bladder system.

One can say that a kind of living, dynamic power – the pulling and pushing behind the breathing process – takes place beneath the diaphragm, where the kidneys and the bladder act and work. This is the first thing we need to bring to our attention when considering the Silver King. The Mixed King (related to the lung) depends for his existence entirely on the other three. For breathing he depends entirely on the Silver King.

Now we can proceed further and ask ourselves: from where does the kidney derive? When we spoke about the lung, we mentioned that it originates in the intestines; it buds out from the intestinal tract. So does the liver. The liver is in this sense derived from the intestine. The lung develops from the upper part, and the liver from the middle part of the embryonic intestinal canal. The origin of the kidney is quite different. The kidneys originate from quite other regions – and I say regions, because among the four organs the kidney is the only one that originates not from one but from two sources.

The kidney arises both from above and from below. It is not that these two grow together in such a way that the one rises and the other falls or sinks down. The power of the bladder in its sucking activity is so strong that it pulls the kidney down step by step, and later on it pushes it up again, as it were. The kidney itself belongs more or less to part of this sucking power from below.

When we study the embryology of humans and higher animals, the whole tragedy of the kidneys begins to be revealed. What were the kidneys before they sank below the diaphragm? They started life high up in the region of the ears, as a series of tiny tubules that then join with the pronephric duct or pronephros. If we pursue the evolutionary origin of the pronephros, we are led through the study of comparative morphology into the very special kingdom of the fish, into the region where the fish breathe by way of gills.

So we then discover that originally the kidneys were organs capable of drawing the living power of oxygen from the water. Now compare such a statement with what Rudolf Steiner said about oxygen in the Agriculture Course. There he says that in the air that we inhale, living oxygen is devitalised, as we would faint if we were to take in living oxygen. Within such a statement, the whole background history of the kidney is contained.[1]

In former times there was no such thing as dead oxygen – it was all alive. When human beings were still floating in the primeval atmosphere of the earth, oxygen was alive, and breathing and eating – breath and food – were part of the same process. At that time the pronephros in the region of the ear took in living oxygen. But gradually, and especially as a result of the Fall, human beings had to descend into solid substance and had to incarnate into matter. This incarnation process was led by the kidneys. The kidneys, which began as organs that took in the living etheric power of oxygen, were more and more compressed into the depths of the developing and evolving material substance of the human organisation.

If we could try to identify ourselves imaginatively with fish, we might experience how fish breathe through their gills and in so doing, listen in to the full extent of the life, being and etheric power pervading the surrounding water. All the oceans of the globe are open to them. The kidneys, in the form of the pronephros of primeval times, listened in to the cosmic powers that were forming, streaming and weaving throughout the entire primeval albumen atmosphere of that time. Animals were formed. Plants acquired their form and dissolved it again. The music of the spheres resounded throughout all this activity and the kidneys heard it. The kidneys brought it about that all the surrounding substances streamed into this floating, very subtle, thin physical organisation of the original human prototype.

Then came the Fall and thereby the kidneys moved downwards. They first appear as the mesonephros. The present mesonephros recapitulates their first manifestation after the Fall. At a later stage, still further down, they appeared as the metanephros. This is the actual form from which the kidney in humans and in the higher animals is derived. In the embryo you can still observe how, out of the bladder, the metanephros rises up. You can feel the serpent power, pulling the kidneys down and uniting itself with them.

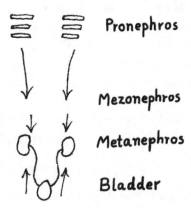

Rudolf Steiner in one of the lectures pointed to a fact that supports what I have just attempted to describe here.[2] He said that in humans the ureters started to develop at the time when, in the outside world, the snakes were evolving. So what is outside was inside, and what is inside was outside. This is the tragic history of the kidneys. If you study the morphology of the ureters, you will see that where they join the kidneys, the head of the snake divides into several heads, turning into the calyces.

We are immediately reminded of the beast which is described by John in the Book of Revelation (12:3), the dragon with seven heads, seven crowns and ten horns, which appears there. We carry this within us, because we carry within us the whole history of human development on earth.

The next question is, how does the kidney carry out its new function? Once it was the ear that listened to the ocean being of primeval earth existence. There it heard the symphony of creation. Then it fell. It dived down into the lower regions of existence. There are many stories that have come down to us about mermaids. There is a wonderful poem by Goethe, 'The Fisherman,' which is a poetic description of what has happened with the kidney. In this poem, it is a mermaid who gradually pulls the fisherman down into the depths. One has to develop a fine sense for such details when attempting to penetrate to the essential nature of the organs.

Now I would like to describe how the kidneys carry out their function. It is wonderful to see how the structure reveals the function, as it does with every organ: From the abdominal aorta, through which blood is streaming in, a small arterial blood vessel arises, enters the kidney and divides into a million convolutions of tiny capillaries or glomeruli.

Each is so small that the single structure can barely be seen with the naked eye. Venous capillaries eventually arise. They converge in very small venous blood vessels which then stream back into a larger vein. There is initially a spreading and finally a renewed convergence within the inner structure, towards the outer boundary. The functional unit is a nephron. About a million nephrons constitute one kidney, so that we carry in us about two million such organelles.

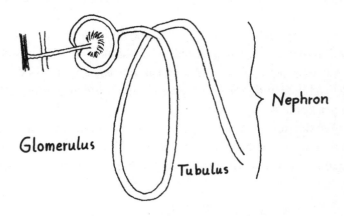

The glomerulus at the beginning of each nephron is surrounded by a cup-shaped formation called Bowman's capsule.[3] This is situated at the closed end of each nephron, which you must imagine as an invagination of the blood, within which the glomerular capillaries are contained. From then on, this structure is called a glomerulus. From there, in a very complicated way, the tubuli of the kidney extend, which finally lead into the central calyces, thus merging with the ureter.

You can see how different this structure is morphologically from the structure of the organ of the lung. In the kidney, the glomerulus is invaginated inside Bowman's capsule. The power of the blood has become much stronger than in the lung; whereas, in contrast, the capillaries surround the alveoli in the kidney; it has become part of the whole organ. It is not like the lung, which tries to find the blood and to incline towards the ear of the blood. In the kidney, the power of the blood has asserted itself. It has invaginated Bowman's capsule, where the renal tubule originates. This is a very similar structure, anatomically, to what we find magnified in the form of the human eye. The eye is built in essentially the same way. What once 'listened' to the creative forces in the primeval atmosphere of the earth now has turned into a 'looking into' the ocean of the blood. With a million little eyes the kidney is forced to look into the blood. What once was outside has turned inside. What was once the ocean of the globe has now become the invaginated sea of blood within us, and into this sea of blood the kidney looks. We should learn to experience this as a visual activity, a seeing activity, through which the manifold physiological functions of the kidney are performed.

We can now ask ourselves what these functions are. Of course it is quite impossible to describe them all in detail, as this would require a very long time to cover thoroughly. We can, however, at least begin to form a preliminary picture of these different functions.

The functions of the kidney are, generally speaking, different from the functions of the liver, and altogether different from the functions of the lung or the heart. If we would learn to see the kidney lovingly, we would need to realise that it is condemned to an existence of continual excretion. The liver is capable of both building up and destroying. But even as it builds up and destroys, nearly all the substances concerned remain within the body, within the whole of the human organism. The kidney is ultimately condemned to excrete, to eliminate. The kidney creates and builds up only to a minor degree. To a much greater degree – I would say to about 70% to 80%, the kidney excretes. The kidney receives the solutes in the blood and subsequently maintains the necessary internal environment of the blood through the activity of the tubules.

Life depends on maintaining a healthy balance of constituents in the blood, on the very many substances contained in the blood serum being present in the right proportions. Our ability to remain conscious and mobile, the ability of our 'I' to have a certain grip on the blood, and of our astral body to work as it should – all this depends upon the level of the blood urea. Much depends on the uric acid content of the blood, the phosphorus content of the blood, the blood sugar level, the different kinds of proteins, albumins and globulins within the blood, and on the distribution of potassium, sodium, calcium and so on. This chemistry needs to be maintained within very precise ranges and relative proportions.

If we were to live according to the exact proportions of the blood constituents, at least some order would be established here on earth! The kidney is the organ that is permanently condemned to regulate the disorder that we create within ourselves. We should increasingly learn to understand this. We depend upon the quality, on the power of discrimination, of the kidney. Through our temperament and moods, through the limitations imposed by our human condition here on earth, our conscious life continually disturbs and potentially undermines our bodily nature. The kidney continually balances, heals and regulates this again. The kidney is like a good mother who runs after her children, cleaning up their mess. Through the natural egotistical tendencies of our psychological makeup we are entirely dependent on the compensatory goodness of the kidneys.

The kidneys are like the galley slaves who were once fettered to the oars of the boats. Day and night they had to pull the boat through the water. The kidneys are such slaves, and we are the ones who misuse them, who are compelled to misuse them; we simply cannot help it. We are born into this earth existence and consequently are bound to continually defile the divine structure and the temple that is entrusted to us. The kidneys do not mind. Please do not think that they feel sorry for themselves. They are represented by the Silver King. They accomplish their task, and they do it with a regal gesture, because they recognise its necessity. For this reason, when the Silver King asks, 'Will my kingdom end?' the Old Man replies, 'Late or never.'

What does the kidney do? How does it accomplish it? First of all, the kidneys keep not only the blood, but all the fluids of our organism in balance through the excretion of urine. If there is too much they excrete more, if there is too little they excrete less. When we are perspiring excessively, we excrete much less urine than if we are not perspiring at all. But the balance of water, of the bodily fluids, does not depend only on the kidneys. Water is, so to speak, an independent entity; it can leave the body through the mouth, the nose, and many other doors and windows, but if that is not sufficient, there is always the exit route via the kidneys. The kidneys always respond to environmental irregularities and threats.

This is the first function of the kidneys. It cannot be said that one function is more important than another; we can only enumerate them all. The second function of the kidneys is a regulatory one, whereby all excess minerals in the body are excreted. This is an act of balance. Sodium, potassium, and so on, are either excreted, or else reabsorbed into the bloodstream. In the kidneys there are the glomeruli. The single functional unit or tubule is called the nephron, which means kidney. In the glomerulus, the drops of filtrate are separated from the blood. They gather together and flow along the tubules, to the calyces, and from there (via the ureter) into the bladder. What is excreted initially is tested – or rather tasted – as it flows along this tubule, so that what is 'looking' in the glomerulus is transformed into 'tasting' in the tubules. But the tasting again requires an active process. If too much of one or another substance has been excreted into the glomerular filtrate, it is registered in the tubules, and the substances concerned are greeted with, 'Hello, dear friend! Back you go.' And back it goes into the blood. You see, this is a living capacity of the kidney to regulate the flow, or surplus, of substances between eye and tongue. This concerns particularly mineral substances such as calcium, magnesium, potassium, sodium, phosphorus, sulphur, and so on. This is the second function of the kidney.

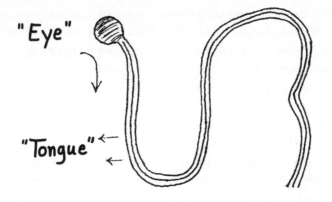

The third function is equally vital among the functions performed by the kidneys. It involves the maintenance of the balance between acids and alkalis within the body, as well as in the serum. If we eat too much protein, we excrete more acid substances; if we eat too many vegetables and become too alkaline, we excrete more alkaline ions.

Then there is yet a further function, which even gives the kidney the possibility of creating a new substance. Within its own realm, it forms ammonia from the waste products of the body's proteins. Although the proteins come to the end of their function after being separated out, the form their excretion takes is via the formation of ammonia and other nitrogenous substances connected with nitrogen radicals. There is one thing here which points to the kings. The kidneys create a substance called renin.[4] This is a substance in its own right, a substance that does not exist in nature, but is built up uniquely by the kidney itself. The kidney attains its sovereign inner autonomy through synthesising renin. Renin is secreted into blood vessels, and its effects radiate into the whole of our body, thereby regulating the tonus of all blood vessels. The tonus of the blood vessels, whether they are too constricted or too relaxed, whether they are active or passive, depends on renin.

Renin is, of course, also an excretion product, a product of

311

metabolism corresponding to the process of ash formation – in the alchemical sense – and concealing a hidden reality within it. Rudolf Steiner frequently pointed to this hidden reality when he spoke about kidney function. Here we come close to the core of the matter regarding this organ. The kidney is the organ that descended from above, leading us into the Fall, giving us the possibility to breathe oxygen, not the living but the dead form of oxygen. Thereby it enables us to have daytime consciousness. We no longer faint, because the kidneys have helped us to eliminate the living oxygen from the atmosphere. Oxygen is now dead, but the atmosphere has become transparent and we are able to see the outer light. In the light of sense existence, the form of all created nature is revealed to us. Just as the outer light appeared around us when we attained our waking consciousness, so the kidney has become the organ through whose deeds inner light can be created. The kidney is the originator, the creator, of this inner light; described by Rudolf Steiner as radiating of the kidney.[5] This *Nieren Ausstrahlung,* as he called it, is like a northern light, not in the form of electricity, but in the form of pure light, coloured light, which radiates out, enabling the astral body to integrate itself into bodily nature.

Once the kidneys had a listening function through which they were able to incorporate living oxygen. Through the Fall, oxygen became dead, human consciousness awoke, light appeared around us, and the kidneys descended in order to become the bearers of the Fall in us. At the same time they became the creators of an inner form of light.

Perhaps it can be pictured like this: in the depths of our body the kidneys are bound to the bladder, and thereby also to our sexual organs. But above, light appears, and with this light the possibility of pure thinking is given to us. Something has fallen; the Silver King has accepted his destiny. But something has been retained, and into this vacant space the lung has entered and united with the kidney. I hope you will understand if I write Eve here, and Adam here, constituting a kind of destiny that is imprinted into our existence. Rudolf Steiner called the lung a representation of Isis. We can also say Demeter, the earth mother. And the kidneys bear the destiny of Adam. The kidneys impart to us what Rudolf Steiner called the dullness or lack of imaginative vitality of our thinking.[6]

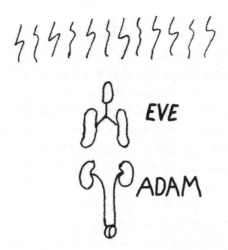

The lungs with the larynx the kidneys with the bladder above.
Right above inner light appears.

Are we now able to find the intuition out of which the kidneys were formed? This takes us back into the realm of Lucifer, and of course to the realm of light. The kidneys need to accept something, in the same way that the surface of the lung must accept our hardened thoughts, and the surface of the liver our comfortable thoughts filled with sentiment. The kidneys become heavy through the need to accept and to bear everything that has become habit during our lifetime.

Just imagine what this means – that one organ has to bear the brunt of all our routines and habits from morning till night! We know how much we depend on our habits: how a pillow must be placed in a certain position before going to bed, how we depend on having a particular kind of food, how our bed needs to be placed at just this angle in the room, how we always put a certain number of cigarettes in our packet in the morning if we are not to become restless, or how we need a particular kind of fountain pen. What accumulates through this habitual junk that we continually gather around us is borne at a cosmic level by the kidneys.

On the other hand, this power to contain, to discriminate, to recycle and to excrete, the sum total of this inner power represents a tremendous force. This force becomes transformative between one life and the next – in the next life our temperament develops out of the habits of our former life. It is the Silver King who has to carry this transformation. He does it with grace and in beauty, but he is obliged to do it. However, if that power already streams up into consciousness in this life – just as it can do for the lung in the form of fixed ideas or for the liver as hallucinations – then from the kidneys all manner of excitement, anxiety and restlessness appear in the soul. Such disturbances then come to expression across a broad spectrum of intensity ranging from more common mild anxiety neuroses to full schizophrenic psychoses. Such tendencies arise either when this power itself is too strong or when the organ's capacity to contain this power is not equal to the task.

We can now appreciate the importance of being able to regulate the forming of our habits, especially nowadays in our anxiety-provoking times. As soon as a habit is broken, a kind of vacuum arises. Fear, stress or restlessness may then overcome someone whose earthly 'I' is not sufficiently robust to endure an hour that is not filled with some kind of habitual activity. We have to become aware of this tendency in order to gain insight into ourselves, and I am sorry to say that on this point those present in this room should not feel excluded. We all suffer continually from such tendencies!

What physical disease of our time is specifically related to the kidneys? It is another condition that has assumed almost epidemic proportions, and is usually described as hypertension. Suddenly blood pressure rises, maybe up to 200 or possibly even higher. The affected person is usually unable to sustain this tremendous tension for long. This is a sign of the Silver King raising his head above the parapet because our production of renin has overtaxed his resources. He is unable to prevent its production. His warning is, 'Do not defile the garment too much which you have been given, because I am unable to keep up with my laundry work or to wash clean what you have soiled.'

Although with this concluding remark I am expressing myself in a humorous way, you will understand that behind my words there is a serious intention. It is a way of coming closer to an understanding of this organ's task and being. We can really only begin to do justice to understanding the cosmic powers which are living in us and which, thanks to Rudolf Steiner, we may now begin to recognise in their full significance and greatness.

Discussion

George Adams: What are the differences between albumins and globulins, and what are their functions in the human body?
Karl König: We usually describe all these substances as protein. The main distinction is between albumin on the one hand and globulin on the other. There are others, but there is no need to go into these for the moment. They are not as prevalent as albumin and globulin. The characteristic of albumin, to put it briefly, is that it is a kind of stabilised protein, a protein that is not easy to dissolve. It is intimately associated with, and becomes the bearer of, several other substances such as gold, iron, lead, tin, and so on. When connecting themselves with living substance, they take albumin as their vehicle. The globulins are much more dynamic, much more in a process of continual becoming. They are easily broken down; they are much more lively. I would not hesitate to characterise them as younger and the albumins as older. In the young child and in the embryo the globulins far outweigh the albumins. As we grow older, the albumins outweigh the globulins.

If we now turn to our main subject of protein formation, we should think particularly of the creation of globulins, which constitute the more cosmic form. The albumins, on the other hand, are connected with the nutrition stream, with oxygen, hydrogen and nitrogen (remember the dynamic process I referred to). There is not yet enough evidence to support this hypothesis, but the character and the form in which the albumins and globulins appear within the blood serum seem to indicate that this is a possible way of accounting for the facts in accordance with present-day knowledge. Dr Husemann has assembled a lot of material bearing this out.[7]

Children with Down syndrome have much larger amounts

of globulins than albumins even in later life. This makes them appear more cosmic, so to speak, and less individualised.

George Adams: When you used the words 'more cosmic,' to which of the two were you referring?

Karl König: I was referring to the globulins. They are the younger, the more cosmic ones. The albumins are the more individualised ones that arise from the nutrition stream.

George Adams: Do I understand rightly that if scientists nowadays employ certain technical terms to identify a number of other kinds of protein, each of these could, according to its character, be assigned to either the albumins or the globulins?

Karl König: That is right.

Question: What about the primary light of which Rudolf Steiner spoke in his lectures to doctors?

Karl König: Rudolf Steiner spoke about primary light in his first cycle of medical lectures; in the third medical lecture cycle, in 1922, he spoke about the radiating of the kidney.[8] However, these two indications are intimately connected. Just this week we have turned again to a verse in *The Calendar of the Soul,* which describes the light – the external as well as the internal one. 'Light from spirit's depths / Strives outward like a sun, ... / And shines into the senses' gloom.' When we follow this up in *The Calendar of the Soul*, we see that there are four verses that relate to each other precisely.[9] These four verses speak about the light, but each time in a different form. We gradually arrive at the following image: The last of these verses in the course of the year – verse 48 – speaks specifically about the light that streams out of the cosmic heights, carrying cosmic ideas into the human soul and awakening within the human heart the power of life. Then, in the cycle of the year, we come to verse 5. There the light is described as a mighty being, which brings the whole creation into existence so that the human being can behold it. Verse 22, which is the counterpart to this one, says the light streams in from outside, bringing fruits within the human soul to ripeness.

The verse of the present week, verse 31, speaks of the light from within streaming out. This is a complete cycle. We can actually see that the light circulates.

Let us start with this week (verse 31). The light is within us. Now, through our sense organs – through the awakening of the summer – the summer of the soul within us streams outwards. After Christmas, at the beginning of spring (end of February and beginning of March), it appears in the heights of the cosmos again, bearing the cosmic ideas (verse 48). It opens up the world of creation. Then, at the beginning of May (verse 5), during the summer, it streams in. The beginning of autumn is marked by a crossing point, which is like the heart of the year. It is this circulation of the light that moves our kidneys.[10]

Comment: You said that the oxygen in our lungs is dead.

Karl König: As soon as you have inhaled, it is already alive, even in the nose, before it reaches the lungs. As soon as it has crossed the boundary of our organism, it is alive. On the outside it can't be, but behind the nostrils, or if you breathe through your mouth, behind the lips, it is already alive. You should not imagine that air streams into the lung nakedly as if we were to breathe directly into the trachea (which happens in the case of an emergency tracheotomy).

Similarly, if you take a sip of water, only a fraction of this pours down the oesophagus (perhaps a third, or if you are very thirsty, one-tenth). It all depends, because the fluid is initially taken up by the gums, by the tongue and by the cheeks, and moves on from there. Certainly the air streams in, and a certain part of it also streams in by way of the trachea, but air is also within us. We are not built like the pictures in an anatomy book, which only show the residual ash of our existence. The air flows in and out. You would never catch a cold if the air only travelled around this passage, because then it would be restrained in its nature. Sometimes the cold wind blows through you and through your whole system, and suddenly your nose is part of the outer world instead of part of yourself. Then it starts to run, because inside, behind the partition, there is life. I mention this because we carry such narrow conceptions around with us, which make us believe that the elements do only what we think they should do. This is not so.

When we are ill, for instance, and our cheeks and our gums are swollen, and everything is inflamed, then the air cannot be absorbed by these walls. Then it simply streams in and streams out again, but usually it takes our astrality in and out with it. Don't mention this to a scientist, of course; he would consider you beyond help! But it is a fact nevertheless. You experience it for yourself that the astral body moves in and out. This is not an exaggeration.

It is the same with the earth. The oxygen underneath the earth is quite different from the oxygen above the earth. With water, it is the reverse – it is more alive above the earth than beneath it.

Question: You spoke of the sunlight as not coming from the sun, but from the light-sphere around the earth. Can you say where the light comes from that affects the plants?

George Adams (who was asked to reply to this question): The other day, Dr König, when you drew the diagram in Lecture 1 (p. 249), you referred to what Rudolf Steiner said about how the light sprouts and grows. If I had been making the drawing, I don't know that I should have put in any arrows. But if I had, I would have made them sprout and grow downwards and not upwards. I have the feeling that the light sprouts and grows towards the earth.

In some of his early lectures, when Rudolf Steiner was speaking in an esoteric mood and context, he used a certain sequence, saying that the plant lives by the *mineral* light, just as man and animal ultimately get their food from the plant. We know that the plant owes its life to the assimilation of the light through the green leaves. You will, no doubt, be familiar with this. Yet, as far as I remember, Rudolf Steiner said that the plant does not live by the primary light, but by the light that is reflected by the mineral kingdom. I think that is a very important point.

Now let us take quite seriously what Dr Steiner said in the lecture to which Dr König was referring.[11] Here is the atmosphere. Then around the earth there is the mantle of warmth, and then further out, actually reaching much farther out, is the sphere of original, primal light. Rudolf Steiner said that this is where the light comes from. It doesn't stream *as light* from the sun. I believe that we have to think of it as follows. The light is the body of the Spirits of Form. You were speaking this morning about the radiating of the kidney. Whether we consider it to be the original, primal light in the microcosm of man, comparable to the primal light that envelops the earth, as described in the 1920 lectures, or whether we think of it as the formative radiating of the kidney, as described in the 1922 lectures, we nevertheless see in it the activity of the Spirits of Form, who bring about the formation of our organs, enabling us to exist in the physical world. Are we not formed in the physical world and for earth-evolution by the Spirits of Form? Their body and instrument is the light.

Now if we speak as scientists, it is very easy, it is very understandable, it is in a way almost necessary for us as scientists to say that the light streams out from the sun. We only need to look at a parasol, and you see that in order to shade yourself from the light of the sun you have to put up the parasol in a certain position. It is quite obvious that the light streams from the visible sun, but it is obvious only as long as you place the shadow-thrower there, and in no other way.

As to what emanates from the sun in the whole of the spatial cosmos, I can think of it as follows. The visible sun is merely the focal point for an activity emanating from the periphery of the entire spatial cosmos. In fact, the entire spatial cosmos depends on the presence of the sun. See what Rudolf Steiner said about this in Dornach immediately before the Agriculture Course.[12] In that spatial cosmos, which is sun-created, the forces of the universe spiritually pour in towards the visible sun, so that it becomes a focus. At this stage it is still an entirely spiritual process and not visible to the physical eye. It is the invisible spiritual light, the light that the mystics seek, rather than external sunlight. Mystics of former times would shut themselves up in their monastic cells and seek to experience the light that no physical eye can ever see. For them, this represented the first of three steps on the mystic path.[13] It is the light of the spiritual sun, which creates the spiritual organism of the entire solar system, the entire planetary system, to which the earth also belongs.

The earth is a brother-sphere of the sun. Earth and sun are akin to each other. Separated, according to Rudolf Steiner, in the Hyperborean Age of earth evolution, they will come together again at some future time. They have never lost their kinship. Now, in the sphere of 'original light' around the earth, there springs the light that eventually becomes visible light. In this visible light – light as we experience it on the physical plane – the spiritual structure of the entire cosmos becomes a spatial form, which we experience as the whole solar system, with all the planets and the sun and moon and the fixed stars and constellations. That is in reality a spiritual structure and at the same time the spatial form of the heavens as we see them physically. As we project our earthly geometry out into the cosmos, it all appears to be beautifully confirmed, down to the very last calculation. It is confirmed from this point of view, and everything seems to say, 'Yes, your thinking is exactly right, and this is precisely how it is.'

Yet it is one enormous 'construct', if we may use this word. It is the great *maya*, for *maya* means nothing but a construct. We now have to become aware that this construct is relative. It is not absolute, it is *maya* – a *maya* filled with wisdom – but which we must nevertheless go through, without becoming imprisoned in it.

So there is no contradiction in asserting that the light springs and sprouts in that sphere surrounding the earth. It is no contradiction if in the sphere of light, as it becomes visible, the appearance arises which shows us the spatial picture of the sun, the picture of Venus, of Mercury, of the constellations. In the rhythms of the cosmos everything behaves in an ordered way, creating a wonderful cosmic geometry for our experience. Yet it only comes into being in that form in the sphere of the earth. The earth-sphere is touched by the influences of the spiritual sun. Then it grows into form, just as our organs grow into the forms that correspond to the archetypal pattern of the human physical body, and also in accordance with the spiritual formative and life forces of which we have been hearing.

Question: Can you say something more about animal and vegetable proteins? What do they represent for us in our food? Dr Steiner said that they are mutually destructive. I wondered whether this means that they destroy each other in our digestion. *Karl König:* Everything that we take in has to be broken down. You know how Rudolf Steiner once drew the ladder of the organic kingdoms – plant, animal, man – in connection with the protein substances which we eat. He said if we break down plant proteins, we have to do it in two steps. First, we have to take it to the animal and then to the human level. If we take in animal proteins we only have to take one step.

I have the impression that what Rudolf Steiner meant by saying that they are incompatible, is simply the fact that as soon as we take in foreign protein, it acts as a poison. It immediately destroys our blood plasma. We should always be aware of the fact that whenever we speak about protein in the blood serum we are referring to the protein in the blood serum around the cells. Within the cells the protein is no longer as important as it is in the blood serum, because there the blood serum is still living substance. There it is being used by the human being himself.

When Rudolf Virchow brought the cell into the foreground of all living existence, he actually excluded the soul and spirit. If you go into the cell (and I say this in connection with what I said about the proteins), you are already in a region of the human organism, where the 'I', in the sense of an I am – no longer has any say, not even via the astral body. Our cells are not the bearers of our individual being. The blood is. The fluids of our body are. But as soon as we are within the cell, we are already in a cosmic sphere, where our ether body can work and live according to its own nature, but where we ourselves are not present.

This may be difficult to grasp from the geometric point of view, but every cell has an inside, so to speak. This inside no longer has anything to do with us. This inside is a cosmic space. Therefore it is as if you had a cell here, and then within the cell you have the nucleus. The nucleus is a cosmic image. It is mainly (I say mainly) the moon. If the cell breaks up – as when the cell divides – it breaks up into the different forms, which in turn reflect the movements of the planets. But we, our protein, our albumin, our globulins, we are in the larger area encompassing the many individual cells; the cell is not us, yet it maintains us.

Karl König (in answer to another question): Low blood pressure is usually associated with a failure of kidney function towards the alkaline side; in high blood pressure the failure is more towards the acid side.

Question: What kind of habit makes the blood pressure rise or fall?
Karl König: On the first evening I spoke of the four meteorological organs and referred to the remark that Rudolf Steiner made in connection with the sucking power of the bladder, where he spoke about inner mobility. If we gulp down our food, if we run after everything, get up quickly in the morning, shave, wash, in the awareness that time is pressing, the train is leaving, the car is waiting, then our inner mobility is continually being destroyed. This leads to high blood pressure; first-born children seem especially vulnerable to this.

On the other hand, if we are in the habit of thinking – which happens not infrequently nowadays – 'Oh well, the Welfare State pays anyhow, I can't be bothered,' this attitude leads to low blood pressure, and inner mobility gradually ebbs away. In this case the attitude, 'We could work, but we might just as well drink a cup of tea,' becomes more and more prevalent. All responsibility is shifted on to others. Nobody quite knows who 'they' are, but 'they' have to care for the education of our child; 'they' also have to care for us when we are old or ill, if we don't get on with our wife, or if we are unemployed. This constitutes the disposition of low blood pressure.

Question: About jaundice: Could you tell us a little bit more about the origin of this virus? Are there any indications at all as to the source?

Karl König: We don't know much about it. We don't even know what type of virus it is. Probably it is one of those that continually change their form and function. We don't even know whether it originated in the east or the west. All this still needs to be investigated. There are many ideas – some of them wild fantasies – but to me it seems that viruses in general represent a crystalline form of what once, at an earlier time, was a living entity. When life is no longer permeated by ether, but enters an intermediary state between living and dead, this constitutes a virus. It refers back to a kingdom that Rudolf Steiner described as inhabiting the previous planetary embodiment of our earth – what Rudolf Steiner named the Old Moon stage of evolution, where there were intermediate forms – not only plant-animals but also mineral-plants. This is what virus forms actually represent. As far as the present stage of earth evolution is concerned, they are displaced entities, so to speak, and therefore cause illness.

Question: Might it be possible for scientists to prove the existence of living and dead oxygen?

Karl König: I have the impression that an ordinary scientist would not be capable of it, but that an extraordinary scientist would certainly be able to do so. I am convinced that the difference could even be demonstrated experimentally. If we were to succeed in bringing both living and dead oxygen into a crystalline form the difference would become obvious immediately. If we could find a way of biologically experimenting with living and dead oxygen, a difference could certainly be proved. I am quite convinced of this, although I must admit that I have no idea how this could be done in practice.

6 The Heart

Lecture 6, Monday, November 3, 1958

In this last meeting we will consider the last of the kings, the Golden King. Although I wouldn't say that he is the best, he is nevertheless the Golden King. When considering the heart, however, preconceived ideas in relation to the connection between gold, heart and sun, are better put to one side. One should rather attempt, from an entirely spiritual point of view, to penetrate through to an understanding of the heart organ from first principles.

When the Green Snake enters the cave of the four kings, Goethe clearly describes the Golden King as small in stature. On his head there is a crown of oak leaves. I think it is significant that at the end of the Fairy Tale this wreath of oak leaves plays a prominent part. When it is placed on the head of the Young King, he is told to 'Know the highest.' These remarks should serve to introduce our exploration into the nature of the heart. When we consider that Rudolf Steiner placed the heart among liver, kidney and lung as one of the four protein-forming organs, we should begin by questioning the justification of this. Physiologically and anatomically, the heart is, after all, not an organ, at least not in the usually understood sense of the word. Neither is it obviously a large metabolic organ or gland in the sense of the liver, the kidney and the lung. Although it is true that we generally refer to the heart as an organ, it has a quite separate function; nevertheless Steiner placed it within this group. In fact, the heart is a muscle.

It has a muscular composition, and physiologists refer to it as a muscular organ. However, the word organ is generally understood to mean something entirely different. We therefore have to start by asking ourselves: how did the heart come to occupy its present anatomical position? In order to pursue this question, we must follow its development through the study of embryology.

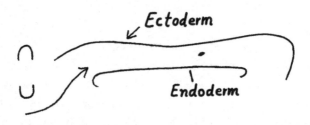

The heart is one of the earliest structures to be formed in the human embryo. It develops almost as early as the primeval organs, such as the primitive gut, etc. Imagine that here we have the first primitive form from which veins, brain, nerves and spinal cord are formed. Here is the primitive gut – the ectoderm and the endoderm – but the heart does not develop within the context of this primitive form. The first seed of the heart actually begins its development outside of it, and only gradually does it develop in such a way that it finds its place between the ectoderm and the endoderm. It must also be born in mind that the heart eventually finds its place between the upper and the lower part of the developing human frame. In more primitive vertebrates, in fish, frogs and even in reptiles, one can observe that the heart lies behind the upper part of the chest, below the throat. Not only is it located higher up, but also exactly in the centre, across the median line. It is situated in the place where our larynx is located.

Certain deductions can be made from this, but I don't want to go too far into this topic, because it would lead us away from what we need to discuss this morning. The main point I wish to convey is that in the course of evolution the heart has only gradually assumed its present position, moving to the left side of the body and assuming its position on top of the diaphragm, with which it is intimately connected. The axis of the heart runs from behind, above on the right, to below in front on the left. This orientation places it in the centre of three-dimensional space.

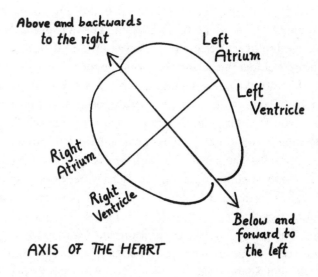

Might we dare to ask how the heart would have been situated had man not gone through the Fall (as described in Genesis) and if the associated Luciferic impact on the development of earth and man had not taken place? From certain indications Rudolf Steiner gave in relation to the anatomy and physiology of the four glands (which we have been studying so intimately) I think we may deduce the following. I would, however, ask you to treat with a certain amount of reservation what I have come to through years of occupying myself with these questions. I simply propose this as one possible way of imagining the primeval morphological human configuration.

It is possible to imagine the development of the kidneys as we did yesterday. It is more or less clear that the kidneys were originally in the upper part of the human body. You must imagine that what I am describing does not refer to physically formed, solid organs, but to a human existence during the time when, according to Rudolf Steiner, the whole atmosphere of the globe was still a kind of primeval milk. This was the primeval albumin, through which human beings were fed, and which at the same time they inhaled.

Probably the liver was in the same place, opposite the spleen, as it is today, only in a different form. Then the lungs formed out of the intestines as a kind of air bladder. This was probably the densest of the structures in this primeval form. In the centre was the heart, holding the balance between the four.

In this morphological configuration, the heart could be likened to the sun among the orbits of the planets. I will draw it to help you to understand it. Here is a sphere, and within this sphere there is a centre. Then the Luciferic temptation took place, and what happened? The kidneys dived down into matter, as a kind of counter-gesture. Rudolf Steiner once described how Yahweh placed the lung in its present position in order to counteract Lucifer's stroke. The further development of the human being led to a very deep disturbance among the organs because each of the organs tried to assume a paramount position. Then Rudolf Steiner told us that one of the pre-earthly deeds of Christ was to restore order within this disrupted activity of the human organs with the help of Krishna. The heart is intimately connected with this process of restoration at that time.

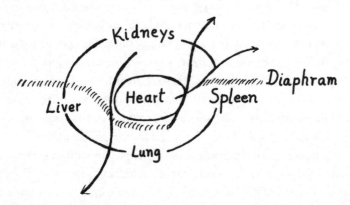

And so the heart moved into the position it occupies today. The diaphragm came about as a result of this, the spleen had to move below, and the heart took over the spleen's former place. So now we have this arrangement.

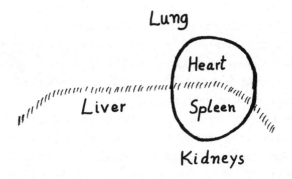

The diaphragm then divides the upper from the lower areas, which was not the case before. The diaphragm is a recent morphological development. It is not present in all vertebrates.

In order to understand the heart, not only in its position, but also in its function and its true being, we would have to consider the other counterpart to the heart, namely the spleen. The spleen represents the unconscious being of the heart. It is impossible to understand the heart – and I mean this literally – without taking into account our unconscious existence; without this we are unable to understand our conscious existence. The spleen, like the heart, is an organ in which part of the bloodstream has been encapsulated. Some of you will remember how important it was to Rudolf Steiner to discover the true nature of the spleen. He spoke about a provisional interpretation of its function in 1911, and later advised Lili Kolisko to carry out particular laboratory experiments on this organ.[1]

The spleen remains a *magnum mysterium* even to this day, although medical science has arrived at many new insights during the last twenty years. Many riddles still need to be solved, however, before a comprehensive understanding of spleen's function can be achieved. The spleen is like a swamp, into which the splenic artery leads the blood. Out of this swamp or pulp comes the splenic vein. Yet if we study the spleen more closely, with all its possible functions, we gradually come to understand that the flow of blood in the spleen can also be reversed. Blood can flow in through the vein, and the artery can lead the blood out again. It has, so to speak, retained a characteristic of a primitive heart, which can reverse its action as required. In this sense the blood flow in the spleen has some resemblance to that in a primitive heart, where blood may also flow backwards and forwards.

If we take one further step, it will become apparent that the heart has not only taken up the earlier anatomical position of the spleen, but that the heart and the spleen together act in conjunction with the blood. This may be understood in the following way. The spleen has mainly to do with the chemistry and the life ether working in the blood; the heart, on the other hand, is concerned with the warmth and the light within the blood. These upper and lower ether forces connected with the blood – this designation is not intended to imply moral judgment – have now become distributed in a different way compared with their configuration during former stages of evolution. The spleen's activity has in consequence become bound up with the sphere of the liver.

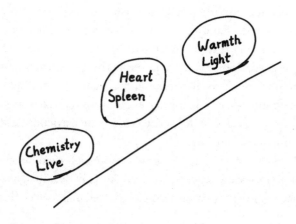

Since 1920, science has coined the term hepatolienal system. This refers to the liver-spleen or hepato-splenetic system, acknowledging that in some respects both organs function together. Occasionally Rudolf Steiner also referred to the unity of spleen and liver. The microscopic anatomy and histology of spleen and liver show a special kind of cell that is found only in these two organs. For instance, the metabolism of iron within the blood and other blood constituents are distributed between liver and spleen. The spleen can become a reservoir for iron, but so can the liver. In pathological situations, spleen and liver are jointly able to produce blood, as normally happens in the bone marrow. One could say that spleen and liver are the 'chemicators' – the life-givers and the life-takers – within the blood system.

Corresponding to the spleen having connected itself with the liver, the heart has connected itself with the lung, together forming the rhythmical system. As you may recall from my earlier remarks, both organs have to do with the oxygen process, whereby digested mineral food is raised up into the etheric sphere. This relationship constitutes one of the pre-earthly deeds of Christ, whereby order was re-established in the human organ structure following the Fall. Because the heart had taken on a new task, this 'unity in duality' of heart and lung came about, and this led to a separation between heart and spleen (the latter organ having been displaced to below the diaphragm).

Thereby the heart also descended. Having relinquished its central sun position and entered the sphere of the three other organs, the heart said, 'Yes, I will become one of you.' When I consider this thought, I always remember how Rudolf Steiner spoke about higher spiritual beings who, in a spirit of sacrifice, renounced their position. For instance, an archangelic being due to rise into the realm of the Archai might renounce this 'promotion' and remain in the lower position in order to take up a particular mighty task in the cosmos. The heart accomplished something that is akin to this process. The heart renounced its key position as a central sun being within the human body.

Thereby it restored balance and order into a realm that had become disordered, thus transforming into a new order what would otherwise have degenerated into chaos. At that moment the heart became a kind of Mercurial or Raphaelic organ. Only in this sense is it really possible to understand why Rudolf Steiner designated the heart as the mediator between the upper (nerve-sense) and the lower (metabolic) functions in the human organisation.

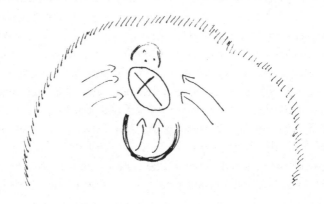

At this juncture we should consider Rudolf Steiner's frequently quoted statement that the heart is a sense organ. What does he mean by this? After all, it falls so lightly from the lips to say that the heart is a sense organ. In a lecture given in Vienna, Rudolf Steiner again described the heart as a sense organ.[2] He describes very precisely how the heart *sees* – he actually uses this word – the entire circulatory system as well as everything going on in the limbs and throughout the metabolic system. Then he goes on to say that through the heart's seeing into the upper part of our organism – and here he specifically refers to the cerebellum or 'little brain' – it becomes aware of the lower metabolic processes. In this way we are able to maintain a state of equilibrium.

Here we have to bear one thing in mind, however. It is not the heart that sees; the heart is really a kind of telescope. It is a kind of living eye-organisation, perhaps even an ear-organisation and a taste-organisation. We are here not dealing with *a* particular sense organ in isolation, but rather with a combination (I don't like the word 'mixture') of these four senses, designated as soul senses by Rudolf Steiner: smell, taste, warmth and sight. It would probably also include hearing. This would give the upper part of the organism the possibility of tasting, seeing, hearing, smelling and monitoring everything that is happening below. Just as the lens is transparent and therefore gives the retina the possibility of receiving light and colour, so the heart, like a lens or cornea, permits the upper part of our organisation to receive, to experience and to monitor what is taking place below.

As soon as we grasp this idea, we can understand why Rudolf Steiner was so frequently up in arms when countering the silly scientific conception that the heart can be regarded as a pump. Nothing, I would say, could be further from the truth than this view of the heart, although assembling a satisfactory body of scientific evidence to underpin this statement is quite another matter.

Now that we can imagine the organisation of the heart as just described, where all the senses by which we normally experience the surrounding environment are combined, I would like to introduce another remark of Rudolf Steiner's. When speaking to physicians he said about the heart: If I look into the world outside and behold the universe, where is it actually to be found? It is to be found within. When I look into my own heart, I find within it the whole universe that we are accustomed to perceiving through our sense organs. This means that everything out there that constitutes the sphere of warmth is within, in this very complex, yet wonderful organisation of the heart; the warmth outside and at the same time the warmth inside, that is the heart. Within this warmth is contained the entire sensory potential, whereby the lower existence can be interpreted by the higher one. This enables equilibrium continually to be created. This is the essential function of the heart.

We will now go one step further. We have heard that the lung gives us the form of the skull in our next life; the liver gives us the configuration of our brain within this skull; the kidney gives us our temperamental possibilities; so what then does the heart give us? Rudolf Steiner described how into the heart as a sense organ stream all the activities of our metabolic system, all the activities of our limbs, of our arms and legs, where we go, what we do, and how we do it. All this is enshrined in the heart as in a little treasure chest. All this then passes through the life between death and rebirth and becomes the field of our karma in our next incarnation.

With our present deeds we prepare the karmic conditions and possibilities for our next life. Rudolf Steiner described this in the following way. Through what we have stored up in the treasure chest of the heart – this is really the story of Pandora's box – we bring with us a hunger to fulfil our karma. Rudolf Steiner actually used the word hunger.[3] We are not satisfied until we have met all the people for whom we hunger, whom we long for. The heart sees to it that this is so. If the powers of future karma stream out in this life prematurely, manic phases will result. In this condition people are no longer fully responsible for what they are doing and they may cause disruptions in the lives of those in their surroundings, occasionally even causing their death.

You can imagine what tremendous forces one is dealing with here, these stored-up forces, which shape the karma in our next life. Here we may identify the cosmic power of hydrogen. We find this power almost exactly as Rudolf Steiner described it in the third lecture of the Agriculture Course. It is capable of completely shattering the present existence and leading it back into the universal realm of spirit in such a way that it can return again. In this context we need only point to the term 'hydrogen bomb' to realise how intimately modern trends are linked to these challenging questions and insights.

This vast field has to do with the surface of the heart. The heart has gradually placed itself into the context of the other three organs. Like the surface of the lung, the liver and the kidney, the surface of the heart itself becomes an organ of memory. Here, however, it is not thoughts or sentiments but pricks of conscience which resound. It is the voice of our conscience that is so intimately connected with the surface of our heart. Because the heart is the mediator within the body and as such carries the conscience for all our bodily functions, it is also able to reflect the voice of our spiritual conscience. The two streams encounter one another in the heart.

Through such insights the complex, all-encompassing activity, function and task of the heart begin to become comprehensible. We are able to understand how intimately connected with the heart, through the elements of hydrogen and warmth, are the activities of our own self, our 'I'. The 'I' has united itself with the heart because it once was situated in the centre and has now become the mediator, the Raphaelic organ. Our limbs represent the mercurial part of our existence. And if our limbs increasingly become inactive to the point of lethargy (as has happened during the last fifty years: we tend to drive rather than walk; we no longer move, we sit!), then the generation of inner, individually created warmth will be very much reduced. This implies that deformations within the warmth organisation of the heart are likely to be increasing. I am now referring to what Rudolf Steiner said in connection with the heart as a meteorological organ. You can now readily appreciate why another epidemic has arisen in our time, and that is heart pathology.

We frequently read how this or that person has suddenly collapsed and died following a short illness. Deaths such as these are usually brought about through deformations of the heart. Through the inactivity of the limbs too much strain has been placed on the heart.

In Goethe's Fairy Tale, the Golden King has a conversation with the Green Snake. The conversation goes as follows.

'What is more wonderful than gold?' enquires the
Golden King.

And the Snake replies, 'Light.'

'And what is more refreshing than light?' he asks.

'Conversation,' she replies.

So the dialogue leads from gold to light and to speech or the logos. This may serve as a kind of closing thought concluding what we have said about the heart organ.

Let us now retrace our steps and survey these four organs once again. We see the lung, the representative of Demeter, the earth mother, bearing carbon (black) with the green vein of oxygen. We see the liver, the Bronze King, with the peach-blossom colour of nitrogen, covered with the white veil of hydrogen. We see the Silver King of the kidney and then the heart, which is entirely permeated by hydrogen. We might also, as a kind of final image, remember that this Bronze King, the liver system, which holds the mystery of the origin of the will, is no doubt a Michaelic organ, as the heart is no doubt a Raphaelic organ. We might also learn to understand how behind what the kidneys have to suffer, stands the being of Uriel in the heights. Connected with the lung stand the deeds of the being of Gabriel.

I would rather discourage you from connecting this imagination directly with the four seasons in the way that Rudolf Steiner related these to the four archangels. I would rather suggest that you confine yourselves, at least initially, to this image of the beings of the archangels, the colours, and the kings. I hope this imagination will help all of us to draw a step closer to the understanding of the protein-creating organs and that these few lectures will have served to strengthen our insight in this respect.

Discussion

Question: I would like to ask how the blood is moved around the body.

Karl König: The movement of the blood is not only related to the etheric forces. The movement of the blood is the result of etheric, astral and 'I' forces. All three together make it possible. You will understand this when I say that before the heart becomes active in the embryo, the circulation is already established. The blood flows out of its own power. Everything that is alive moves, and the blood prepares its own channels, its own vessels, in order to be able to move in them. Then the gradual ooze of the blood becomes rhythmical, and the pulsation comes about through the astral body and the 'I'. So the heart, in point of fact, provides the physical context that enables the direction of flow to be established and regulated.

In this complicated re-direction of the flow through the heart, the venous blood coming up from the right is directed into the lung, re-directed back into the body and so on. You must imagine that about five litres of blood stream through the heart every minute. I would like to add something that would have been too much to mention in the lecture. This concerns the temperature of the heart. The muscle of the heart does not move through nervous activity. It is absolutely obvious – and this is also acknowledged by scientists – that the motor activity of the heart muscle is not brought about by stimuli coming from the central nervous system, but that it develops its own driving force from within itself.

Again, in connection with the motor activity of the heart: we can say that the heart consists of four chambers, two auricles and two ventricles. The auricles and ventricles move separately, but this movement is co-coordinated within the heart, and this gives rise to an entirely new, unique organic structure not to be found anywhere else in the body. It is neither a muscle nor a nerve. I am referring to what is called the bundle of His (after the Swiss anatomist Wilhelm His). This bundle of His together with several other structures (the auriculo-ventricular node for example) direct the action of the muscle. This bundle is an amazing organ. It is among the most beautiful structures to be found anywhere in the body. If we look at its form in the right way, it undoubtedly resembles a kind of plant root. Reaching up are two tiny 'leaves', so that suddenly we have a plant starting to grow within the centre of the human – as well as animal – organisation. From this it can also be seen that the heart and the blood manifest their own independent movement.

Question: What about the healing effect of particular plants on certain organs?
Karl König: I cannot give you a definite answer with respect to all the organs, but I would suggest that the Compositae would be valuable for the kidneys, and the Ranunculaceae for the lung. I am doubtful whether any particular plant family would be of special value for the liver. But for the heart, all types of Rosaceae would be helpful. The rose is primarily a sun plant that also has a particular relationship to Mars.

George Adams: The fact that the rose relates to Mars should remind us of an element that is receiving increasing attention and is being used more and more. Perhaps one could say that, very roughly speaking, it has its function and place somewhere between silica and steel. I am referring to titanium. It is known that, among the plants, the rose in particular contains titanium.
Karl König: How interesting! This is most important. I am very grateful for this indication. During the last four or five years it has also been found that cobalt is of great importance for the formation of blood. Cobalt is a trace element. It is contained in bone marrow, and a lack of cobalt leads to serious illnesses. So far

we don't know too much about titanium, but this remark might lead us to certain insights.

George Adams: When I was studying chemistry, I was surprised to learn that titanium was a rare element, but if we roughly list the elements of the earth in order of weight, including calcium, oxygen, hydrogen, titanium is in ninth place. There is an enormous amount of titanium in the earth. There are whole mountains of titanium ore in the earth.

Karl König: Of course I have been able to mention only very little of what Rudolf Steiner said with regard to the heart. In a lecture in 1919 he drew attention to the fact that since the year 1721, the heart has altered its condition.[4] Since that year, the etheric heart has loosened its connection from the physical structure of the heart, and that as a result very great changes in the whole life and existence of humanity have come about. He didn't specify which changes he was referring to, but I have pondered on this, and I have formed he impression that they are connected to the Pietistic movement which arose on the Continent around that time. In England, this movement found its expression in the Wesley brothers.[5] These events could well have been triggered by the changes Steiner was referring to. In the future the heart will continue to alter its whole physical-spiritual configuration.

In his lectures given in 1922, Rudolf Steiner drew our attention to the fact that in the course of our own individual development in childhood, the whole structure of the heart alters.[6] He used the following words: 'the etheric heart that we bring within us from birth gradually withers away and is rebuilt by an entirely new etheric heart.' One day we should bring such things together, but a whole lecture cycle would be needed to do justice to this theme.

George Adams: I think what you referred to as the Pietistic movement, which came to a culmination about that time, found its strongest expression in England through George Fox, the founder of the Quakers. He, in particular, had a spiritual experience connected with the blood and the Christ impulse. He had a direct experience of the Christ light through the blood. At the end of the First World War, when the Quakers were doing so much relief work in Europe, Dr Rittelmeyer took a great interest in them.[7] He became acquainted with some of the leading Quakers, and he asked Rudolf Steiner what kind of movement this was. Rudolf Steiner answered that he did not know, but that he had the impression that it had something to do with the blood.

Karl König: It would be very important, in connection with this remark about 1720, to mention the fact that other significant movements sprang up on the Continent, especially in western Germany. There were some amazing personalities. Swedenborg had his great initiation in London in 1740–42.[8] All this reached a peak around this time. I have always thought that this freeing of the ether heart from its bondage to the physical function engendered new developments, such as a renewed Christian experience, in the people of that time. Bach's music is another example of this.

George Adams: Dr König, I wonder if you could say any more about what Dr Steiner said in his Torquay lectures about the need to 'think with the heart?'[9] In one of these lectures – which you recommended as preparatory reading for this conference – Rudolf Steiner spoke of hydrogen, the heart and the faculty of thinking. Can we connect this with what we have read in the Agriculture Course about the functions of hydrogen?

Karl König: Again, I can only give some indications. I would recommend studying the lecture on hydrogen, which Rudolf Steiner gave in October 1923.[10] Even if you make every possible effort to understand this lecture, you may say, 'My goodness, it is absolutely unintelligible.' Yet because of certain things contained in this lecture, I know that it contains a deep truth.

Rudolf Steiner told the story of the snake. You are to imagine a snake, which produces eggs. Of course in most snakes the eggs are laid outside, so that the cosmic warmth can surround them. The cosmic warmth is needed for the development of the young. But if you take the snake out of its natural environment and withhold water – you know that hydrogen is contained in water – the snake will lose its ability to prepare a new skin, and will go on living in its old rags. At the same time it will also be quite unable to produce the shells for the eggs, and in this way we will have made the snake produce living young the following year. All this is connected with hydrogen. Steiner then went on to describe sodium – sodium carbonate.

I have studied this lecture again and again, and this has helped me to understand many things, with the exception of hydrogen! Still, there is no doubt that hydrogen has the following function. You may soon understand what I mean when I simply describe the facts, without as yet making any connection between them. In his lectures to the workmen, Rudolf Steiner spoke on the one hand about light, and on the other about electricity. By means of light we are able to think. Electricity enables us to carry out our reproductive activity. Then he connected both thinking and reproductive activity with hydrogen. He mentioned that male semen contains a particularly large amount of hydrogen, while in the female ovum there is nothing but protein. It is the hydrogen that stimulates the protein to develop, to divide, to grow and to reproduce.

For this reason we have to see the substance hydrogen in connection with the two activities for which the Old Testament uses the phrase 'to know'. I have the impression that this is a further key to the tremendous question of hydrogen, because here we also have warmth, in one case containing light, in the other containing electricity.

In this lecture Rudolf Steiner made other remarks that can make one's hair stand on end. He said, for example: You know I always speak about hydrogen, but hydrogen is phosphorus and phosphorus is nothing but hydrogen! If we were to study this more deeply, I am sure it would become apparent to us in how far hydrogen and phosphorus are the same. He even said that if our chemistry were developed far enough, we would be able to change phosphorus into hydrogen and hydrogen into phosphorus. This may already be a known fact, but I have not been able to keep abreast of developments in modern chemistry.

George Adams: Rudolf Steiner said that we develop carbon dioxide in our head organisation, which makes us clever and intelligent. Now when observing nature, we discover the following: when organic life decays, hydrogen arises as gas – known as marsh gas – also hydrogen sulphide and phosphine. It stinks terribly! However, in our gut we also develop marsh gas, methane, which stinks and which dulls down our consciousness. Now Rudolf Steiner also said that we take a little of the marsh gas into our head nature, so preventing us from becoming too clever. That is important, because it was mentioned that oxygen brings the light into the physical. In so far as the light of intelligence is brought into the physical, we are clever. Where dullness predominates, intelligence is still present, but it has not been brought into the physical to the same extent. This again has to do with the nature of hydrogen. In the one instance carbon combines with oxygen, forming carbon dioxide, and in the other it combines with hydrogen, forming methane.

Karl König: Here I can add another remark made by Rudolf Steiner in the same lecture. There he says that as soon as hydrogen is combined with light, it becomes good and clever. But as long as it is connected with marsh gas, in the dark, it remains stupid. This means that hydrogen in the darkness and hydrogen in the sphere of light are two different things.

George Adams: Dr König, I am very grateful that, in drawing attention to the hydrogen lecture to workmen, you have pointed to the question of electricity. I think that it is a very important task to find out, from a spiritual point of view, what enables us to hold the balance. We shall never achieve this if we are afraid of electricity or even think that it is something to be avoided.

We have to penetrate this question with our thinking. I think that the picture you have given provides a key. I couldn't help but be reminded of a particular lecture, which has meant a great deal to me. In England we have a number of Steiner's lectures on colour published in one volume, *Colour,* which in the German edition are found separately. Dr König referred to one about peach-blossom, green, black and white. The same volume contains lectures Rudolf Steiner gave on December 5 and 10, 1920. Here he spoke again about colours, and about light and thought on the one hand, and darkness and will (volition) on the other. He also referred to darkness as matter. When speaking about the polarity of light and will, or thought and will, he said, 'Will or, if I gave to what I am speaking of a more oriental colouring, I could also call it love.' When Dr König speaks about the two aspects of knowing – knowing in the biblical sense – we can see both of them in the sphere of cognition and in the sphere of will or of love.

We must have the courage to touch upon this secret. When speaking once again to scientists – mainly physicists – in those two special courses he gave to scientists in Stuttgart, Rudolf Steiner said that in the realm of electricity and magnetism we have the essence of matter. If you seek the secret of matter, you will find it in electricity and magnetism. What Rudolf Steiner said then coincides absolutely with the current scientific findings.[11]

He says that electricity has a direct kinship to what lives in human will. If you consider those experiences that the human being can derive directly on the basis of his will system, you find something that is akin to electricity and magnetism. We find here an intimate network of relationships. We are called upon to find the courage not to run away from the realm of electricity, but to allow Rudolf Steiner to guide us into that secret.

I have been very gratified to hear just now from Dr König, and a few weeks ago from other friends on the Continent, that the recent large medical conference, I think it was last Easter, when doctors and therapists gathered together, addressed current aspects of atomic science and technology.

In conclusion, I would like to add a few words. We have been reminded again and again during these days of the World Conference in 1928 in London.[12] It was almost as though a number of diverse threads which were woven at that event have come together again now in a very particular way. Maurice Wood was there, Carl Alexander Mier and also Dr König were present. I know that this event was a particularly important experience for Dr König and it was for us too.

That World Conference came about through the initiative of Dr Wegman. It was only three years after Dr Steiner's death, and she was there with all her heart forces, and in the confidence that the Michael forces and the healing, therapeutic impulse of Anthroposophia would stream through into the western world. It was Mrs Pease, who then became the president of our agricultural work, who had made available the resources to enable that World Conference to take place. Mr Dunlop too supported it with all his good forces.[13]

Now I would like to say the following: You as farmers and gardeners have asked Dr König to hold this course for us, inspired by the following question: how can the healing forces, how can the medical wisdom Rudolf Steiner developed in conjunction with Dr Ita Wegman come to life in the English-speaking world? It lives in the educational work of the anthroposophical movement; not only in the realm of special needs education, but also in mainstream Rudolf Steiner Schools. It lives in your farming and gardening work too. Yet this impulse, as medical wisdom, has somehow been prevented from entering the English-speaking world. There is something in what we have received during these days that contains the possibility for that hindrance to be overcome.

By holding this in your hearts dear friends, you may consider how you might give something back in support of this impulse. For myself, I feel that the key lies partly in this. What Rudolf

Steiner gave in a Central European language – a Central European language that was able to make anthroposophy, wisdom of the human being, manifest by way of that power of methodical thinking which was at that time the necessary spiritual method in Central Europe – everything he imparted needs in some way to be translated into the kind of understanding and the kind of impulse of the heart that cosmic wisdom calls forth, by a cosmic and religious approach, a cosmological approach, which lives in the English-speaking world. Perhaps the agricultural movement in this country, in the echo that comes from Dr König's lectures, could help to awaken this impulse. This could happen, especially if we carried in our heart the wish that the anthroposophical medical movement in the English-speaking world should prosper and thereby overcome those deep occult hindrances that have stood against it. We can help this to come about, for I really believe that it can, in the near future, and to no small extent through the work that you, Dr König, are doing.

Two Essays

The Relation of Intestine and Brain

Working Paper for the Agricultural Group, October 9, 1964

In the fourth lecture of *Introducing Anthroposophical Medicine,* Rudolf Steiner pointed to an important correspondence. He said the following:

> People ... usually do not consider the fact that the human being manifests as a duality and that anything taking on form down below is always parallel to an organ that appears up above. Certain organs cannot appear in the upper body unless their parallel organs, or counterparts, are able to develop in the lower body. The more the forebrain develops in the course of animal evolution, eventually assuming the form it has in the human being, the more the intestines develop in the direction that leads to storing the remains of food. There is an intimate connection between the formation of intestines and the formation of the brain: if the colon and the appendix had not appeared in the course of the evolution of animals, physical human beings who can think would also ultimately not have been able to appear, because humans have brains at the expense – at the very pronounced expense – of their intestinal organs.

The intestinal organs are the faithful obverse of the structures in the brain. To make it possible for you to be relieved of physical activity for the sake of thinking, you must burden your organism on the other hand with everything that gives rise to the need for a fully developed colon and bladder. This means that the highest activities of soul and spirit in the human physical world, to the extent that it is bound to the full development of the brain , is also bound to the corresponding development of the intestines. This is an extremely significant connection, a connection that sheds a great deal of light on all of natural creation.[1]

From this description it is clear that the development of the form of the brain and of the form of the intestine must be regarded as closely connected. What Rudolf Steiner called forebrain can only be considered as partly the same as the whole pallium. It seems more likely that the small intestine and the large intestine together have convolutions similar to those of the cerebrum, corresponding to the whole neopallium.

The duodenum with liver and pancreas are a parallel formation to the subcortical (cover) and thalamus. The hypophysis is parallel to the gall bladder. The stomach is the midbrain with the attached fourth ventricles and the medulla oblonga. The oesophagus with pharynx are the spinal cord with the spinal ganglion and nerves belonging to it.

So that we have approximately the double figure shown. Here we are first of all concerned with form: with the form of the two polar systems, the intestinal duct and the central nervous system. However, in the Agricultural Course and in other places, Rudolf Steiner spoke of *forces*, rather than of form.

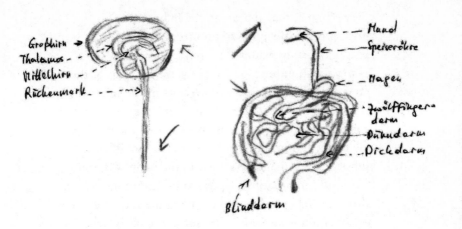

From the original working paper.

Left: Cerebrum, Thalamus,
Midbrain, Spinal cord.

Below: Appendix

Right: Mouth, Oesophagus,
Stomach, Duodenum,
Small intestine,
Large intestine

In the head we have to do with cosmic forces, since the
cosmos is perceived with the senses, which are located
primarily in the head. In the metabolic-limb system, on
the other hand, we have to do with earthly forces; with
cosmic substances, but earthly forces. Just think how
we are constantly engaged with earthly heaviness when
we walk, how in fact everything we do with our limbs is
connected with the Earth.

But the *substances* of the lower organism, which are described
here as cosmic, must not be equated with dung. These are substances that are taken up by the formative forces and used to form
organs such as liver and spleen, also bones and muscle tissue.

Dung, on the other hand, is digested and processed nourishment. We are further told:

Everything ... that appears in the brain as earthly matter, is actually an excretion from the organic process. Earthly matter is excreted in order to serve as a foundation for the ego. Now, on the basis of the process in which foodstuffs are consumed, digested, and distributed by the metabolic-limb system, a certain amount of earthly matter is able to reach the head and the brain, and in this way a certain amount of earthly substance is actually deposited in the brain. But the foodstuffs are not only deposited in the brain, they are also excreted by the intestines along the way ... What is the brain mass, actually? The substance of the brain is simply intestinal content taken as far as possible ...

It would be crass to say that what is present in the brain is simply a more highly developed manure pile, but objectively this is quite correct. The manure is transformed by means of the organic process into the noble substance of the brain, where it becomes the basis for development of the ego.[2]

We therefore have following.

- Above in the nerve-sense system,
- Cosmic form and earthly substance;
- Below in the metabolic-limb system,
- Earthly form and cosmic substance.

In this lower cosmic substance, however, an earthly substratum, manure, is prepared as a preliminary stage of the brain substance. This, so to say, not quite earthly manure is polarised by another process no longer quite cosmic, in the upper organism: thinking as man has developed it. Just this correlation alone provides a first insight in the connection prevailing here.

By the way of a brain built of physical substance, a thinking can develop that inclines toward earthly sense experiences. This actually takes place in the cosmic sense processes that relate to the cosmic nutritional stream.

By the way of an intestinal tract built of cosmic substances, dung is formed through constant excretion. It becomes a material counterform to thinking. It is the first step in the physical development of brain substance, a development that is then carried much further.

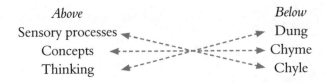

Above ... *Below*
Sensory processes → Dung
Concepts → Chyme
Thinking → Chyle

This is the first chapter toward an understanding of the process picture above.

The Plant-Seeds Are Quickened

In memory of Eberhard Schickler

I

Many of the verses given to us by Rudolf Steiner describe the mysterious dual relationship in which is revealed the weaving between the inner being of man and the world surrounding him. This provides the reader, speaker or meditant of these verses with a mirror, in which one is able to recognise oneself in the process of contemplating the world. One such verse is:

> The secrets of your own soul
> Are revealed in the countenance
> That the world presents to you.
> The inner being of the world
> May be discovered in the countenance
> It imprints in your soul.

In one of his notebooks of 1911 we find the following entry:

> In the boundless outer world
> You may find yourself as human being.
> In your most intimate inner life
> You may sense boundless worlds.

> Thus it is revealed,
> That the solution to the riddle of the world
> Is the human being.

Since that time Rudolf Steiner revealed to us more and more solutions to this riddle, and this process of spirit cognition will progress to the extent that this unique method of cognition is taken up more widely. The key is the need for the human soul to learn to grasp itself in the works of nature, and for the human spirit to find the answers to the riddles of the world in its own soul. The outer questions are led towards inner answers, while inner riddles find their solution in the outer world.

> In the contemplation of nature
> Individual phenomena deserve as much attention as
>   the whole;
> Nothing is merely internal, nothing merely external;
> For what is internal is external.
> So grasp hold without hesitation
> The holy open secret.

Time and again Rudolf Steiner endeavoured to represent this 'holy open secret' in ever new ways in lectures and essays, sketches and paintings, in poems and verses. In succinct words he inscribed this method into the conscience of many people; whole series of meditations are devoted to this 'Janus head'.

> If you would know the world,
> Look into your own soul.
> If you would know yourself,
> Look out into the world.

In the processes of nature are revealed the secrets of the human soul. In the outer world they take the form of images, while in the inner world they become experiences.

The composition of the *Soul Calendar* has been created on the basis of this open secret, and each individual verse is mirrored in this way in its counterpart. To give just two examples: 'The soul's creative power' (Verse 41); 'The world's bright loveliness' (Verse 12).[1]

Here the inner experience of Epiphany is contrasted with the exuberance of St John's tide:

> Can I then the being know
> That, known, it finds itself again
> In the soul's urgence to create? (Verse 35)

> Can I expand my soul
> To grapple to her being
> This word of worlds in germ conceived? (Verse 18)

Here too we find the contrast that opens up between inner and outer, which, however, in the cognitive process does not remain antithesis, but provides the mutual solution to the apparently polar phenomena. Being and world turn into imaginative answers to the questions arising in the soul. The soul, in turn, solves those riddles that emerge in the processes of the sense world and in world existence.

II

'Our' table grace, which is said every day before meals by thousands of people across the whole world, has been condensed out of this open secret. Many children have learnt it, and for a growing community of adults it has become part of their daily bread, just like the food it is referring to. It resounds in large circles as well as where only two people sit at table together; in the family circle as well as in the individual soul. Wherever people partake of a meal and don't merely eat, it has found a place and has become a holy, open secret.

The plant-seeds are quickened in the night of the
    earth,
The green herbs are sprouting through the might of
    the air,
The fruits are ripened by the power of the sun.

So quickens the soul in the shrine of the heart
So blossoms spirit-power in the light of the world,
So ripens man's strength in the glory of God.
(Trans. George and Mary Adams)

This is the form it was given by Rudolf Steiner. The first verse describes an event taking place in nature; the second verse speaks of the inner life of the soul. However, both verses are permeated by a progression carried by the verbs: quickening – sprouting – ripening. One can experience the quickening as a process of unfolding, which finds its continuation in sprouting and finds its rounding-off in the ripening process, becoming ready for harvest. The vowel *'ei'* in the German word *keimen* (quickening) represents an opening process; the same sound in the word *reifen* (ripen) denotes fulfilment. Between the two stands the *'o'* of *sprossen* (sprouting): *ei – o – ei*.

The image of the unfolding plant appears in front of our inner eye in simple but appropriate word pictures. They lead us to a perception of the forces shaping the plant, which are active in the elements: the dark of the earth, the powers of the air, and the might of the sunlight. The plant – the living and shaping 'water', has been formed out of the forces of earth, air and light. The earth bestows firmness, the air wafts through, the light shapes the plants.

Any further indications would be superfluous. The magnificent and marvellous growth process of sprouting, growing and ripening, brought about through earth, air and light, is painted into our souls through the power of the vowels and consonants. It is able to submerge itself in the great laws that govern this process of becoming, and spirit-recollection permeates it. The evolution of the earth, which bears within it the memory of its Saturn, Sun and Moon phases, is active behind this process of becoming, filling it with substance. This image becomes reality, and the person saying this grace experiences himself as part of this process of the world's becoming.

Germinating (or quickening), sprouting and ripening re-appear, but now they are linked to the inner processes of the human soul, describing the process which reveals itself as the 'secret of one's own soul'. The soul quickens in the shrine of the heart; spirit-power blossoms in the light of the world; man's strength ripens in the glory of divine existence.

Here those saying the grace do not experience their past development, but the promise of their future becoming. As they look upon the plant and experience a memory of their earlier existence, so now they look upwards and recognise their higher being awaiting them.

They have been endowed with the shrine of the heart; they find themselves in the light of the world; in the glory of God their true being unfolds. The natural human being gives birth to a divine scion, pointing to the future. The soul quickens, the spirit blossoms, and the higher man ripens in the arms of the spiritual world. We can experience the Christmas mood of the Soul Calendar.

> I feel the spell dissevered
> In the soul's womb freeing the spirit child.
> The holy word of worlds
> Has in the heart's clear light
> Begotten heaven's own
> Which, rising from the god in me
> Goes paeaning to the corners of the world.

Here we find a similar process of enhancement as in the verse above. Soul's womb, word of worlds, the god in me. Yet here

everything is raised to the level of the sacred, elevated and surrounded by the grace of Christmas.

The first verse of the grace points to the polar verse of the
Soul Calendar; in the ripening season of summer the human
being speaks:

> I feel the spirit's weaving
> Spell-bound within the world's array. (Verse 15)

The second verse is the fulfilment at Christmas tide, which
reads:

> I feel the spell dissevered
> In the soul's womb freeing the spirit child.

The praying, speaking, meditating human being moves
between. In the enchanted glory of the senses – experiencing
the plant's unfolding – dim memories of his own spirit past rise
up. Human beings feel their own quickening, sprouting and
ripening reflected in the pace of world evolution. Their own
power of perception, 'conjured free', leads them into their own
inner being, enabling them to intuit their future form. The soul
quickens, the spirit sprouts, their essential human power comes
to manifestation. Manas, buddhi and atman, soul spirit, life spirit
and spirit man bow down and fill man with their promise for the
future of humankind.

In humble gratitude human beings contemplate the unfolding
of the plant, which offers itself up and becomes their food. They
receive the plant in mindfulness of their higher being, which
they are striving to attain in hope-filled courage. They experience
themselves placed between nature and spirit existence. They bow
down and eat, looking upwards, promising themselves that the
transformation of nature can only be effected through their own
devotion, cognition and striving.

What once quickened, sprouted and came to maturity, now

becomes – elevated and spiritualised – the future germ, sprout and fruit of man.

III

There are two other verses which are used as graces before meals, and which have an almost identical-sounding opening line as the one on 'our' table grace. One of these verses reads:

> The plant-seeds spring
> In the womb of earth,
> The sun draws them
> From the darkness
> Into the light:
> So does the good
> Sprout in human hearts.
> The soul draws
> Its striving power
> From spirit grounds.

Here the threefoldness of quickening – sprouting – ripening is missing. Instead, a duality of above and below, of earth and sun is employed. We are confronted with a very vivid image transformation. Outside, the plant-seeds are springing in the womb of the earth; in the inner being of man the good sprouts in human hearts. The sun wakens the plants and draws them towards the light. In the inner being of man it is the soul, which – like the sun – delivers the human 'I' from the spirit grounds of the good germinating in the heart. Here too we encounter the image of the spirit child appearing in the womb of soul.

The second verse – similar to one above – reads:

> The plant-seeds spring in the womb of earth
> And waters rain from heaven's heights.
> So does love spring in human hearts
> And wisdom streams into human thought.

Here we find the same starting point in the first line: the quickening plant in the womb of the earth. Then the image changes, and instead of the radiant light of the sun, it is beneficent rain which is streaming down. In the next line the inner being of man is metamorphosed in accordance with the outer happening. Love springs in human hearts, and wisdom, filling human thinking, streams down.

If we place these different pictures side by side and attempt to understand their language, we find a common theme running through all the verses. The womb of the earth or the night of the earth corresponds to the shrine of the heart in the human being. The various aspects of man's inner life develop in the seclusion of the heart:

> So quickens the soul,
> So sprouts the good,
> So does love spring.

Whether we are children, adolescents or adults, the soul quickens in all our hearts. Every day anew the evolving human soul is revealed in the formation of the human heart. Every awakening in the morning is a renewed quickening of the soul in the ground of the heart. Only when the heart has stopped beating, can the soul withdraw from its earthly existence and cross the threshold to the land of spirit. On earth, however, it perpetually quickens in the heart.

Because the soul is able to quicken in the heart, it is able to transform into light. When the human heart's transformation into light takes place, the soul becomes an inner sun, which quickens the good in the heart. The good in turn awakens those spirit powers which are able to allow the wisdom of the world to stream, enabling love to arise in the human heart. This is why we are able to read in the Soul Calendar:

> In the light that wills from heights of worlds
> To stream amain into my soul,
> May sureness of world thinking
> Shine out, to solve the riddles of the soul,
> Massing the power of its rays
> And waking love within the hearts of men. (Verse 48)

Now the images of the three verses condense and flow together into a single one: the soul quickens in the heart; it becomes like the sun and receives the human 'I' from spirit depths. The good is able to quicken in the heart; it grows and calls down the wisdom of cosmic thinking from the heavenly heights; this streams down like rain, awakening love in the heart.

A new spirit physiology of the heart organ begins to be revealed here. The heart is likened to the earth. Just as on the earth all life is formed, the plants are quickened, grow and fruit, so the human soul is quickened in the dark space of the heart's shrine. Here the good and eventually love is awakened, for in the heart a similar process takes place as it does on the earth. The heart too is to become a sun.

> Therefore the sun
> In the human cosmos
> Is the heart;
> Therefore in the heart
> The human being
> Is closest to his own being's
> Deepest source.

IV

A grace said before a meal is not really a prayer, but rather a blessing for the persons about to partake of a meal as well as for the food itself. The verse 'Christens' the food, as it were. The person about to partake of it enters a reflective mood, engendering consciousness of his divine origin. The higher powers are called upon not only to grant the food as nourishment but also to make it beneficial. An often-used table grace asks:

> Father, bless this food
> For our strength and to your glory.

Or:

> Come, Lord Jesus, be our guest
> And bless the food you have granted us.

Blessings of this kind are still being said at many tables where food is eaten in the sight of the Godhead. Such verses, however, are still imbued with a certain personal-egotistic motif. Human beings pray for divine blessing so that the food may benefit them. They are mindful that the food is bestowed on them by the hand of God, and almost as a matter of course they remember the lines from the Lord's Prayer:

> Give us this day our daily bread.

Even the Bushmen pray: 'O Cagn, O Cagn! Are we not your children? Do you not see our hunger? Give us nourishment!' And the Ainu pray: 'O you great God reigning above the waters, O Water God, we are now going fishing. Pray grant us many fishes.'[2] These prayers too are a supplication of the Godhead, arising from the request for the granting of the daily bread and for beneficial effect on the person who will eat it.

In the course of human evolution – through the entry of the Christ into the earthly world and the enactment of the Mystery of Golgotha – a new understanding arises for the significance of the meal. A sense for the mystery of the feeding arises and finds expression in that eloquent verse by Angelus Silesius, entitled: 'Man does not live by bread alone':

> 'Tis not the bread that feeds us; what feeds us in the bread
> Is God's eternal Word, is Spirit and is Life.[3]

This verse is imbued with the clear sense that God himself – his word, his life and his spirit – are present and active in every kind of food. Thereby every meal is elevated to the level of the Eucharist. A similar verse by Rudolf Steiner, which can be used as a table grace, was given to me many years ago by a friend.[4] It fits into this 'Eucharistic' group of blessings:

> May you, O higher life
> Be thanked by our life,
> That its body
> Through your body
> May be nourished.

What once was a blessing now becomes transformed into knowledge of the continual presence of God in the bread. From a request for help and blessing – for the hunt and the prey, for nourishment and food – a consciousness has developed for the fact that all matter, according to the theologian and pupil of Zinzendorf, Friedrich Christoph Oetinger, is the 'end of the paths of God'.

The *new* table grace, however, is neither supplication nor prayer for blessing, nor is it solely an awareness of the Eucharist. It places human beings themselves in a position of mediator in such a way that they are able to unite the world of nature created by God with the spiritualisation of their own soul. In this way human beings become the executor of a cosmic communion, which in and of itself constitutes a sacred and therefore healing form of cognition. They see themselves as beings living in the house of nature. At the same time they are mindful of the spirit path of their soul, which is revealed through the image of the processes of nature.

While in the earliest periods of human history blessings were said in mindfulness of the Father God, the meal transformed into the Eucharist is partaken of in the name of the Son. Where human beings begin to be mediators between nature and soul-spirit, we have the beginning of the age of the Holy Spirit.

V

'Our' table grace opens the door to this new realm. It should be said with devotion, as devotion is the virtue of the consciousness soul. According to Rudolf Steiner, the consciousness soul will never gain an understanding even of an external matter unless it is approached with love and humility, for our soul passes by the things it does not approach with love and humility, or, in other words, with devotion. Here our attention is drawn to a cardinal virtue, which human beings need to develop in our time.

In a lecture on the mission of reverence, humility and love are described as the two wings of this gate of the soul. 'Love is one part of reverence and devotion is the other.'[5] Both feelings lead the consciousness soul to the gate of the spiritual world. Thinking alone is incapable of accomplishing this.

> This quality of will, which enables people to wish to carry out their aims with regard to the unknown, is devotion. While the will can supply devotion to the unknown, feeling can become love of the unknown, and when the two combine together they give rise to reverence in the true sense of the word. Then when reverence arises, as the mutual fructification of this and devotion, it will become the driving force that will lead into the unknown in such a way that thinking can grasp it. Thus, then is how reverence becomes the educator of the consciousness soul.[6]

The table grace we have received from Rudolf Steiner enables us to practice devotion every day. The first part teaches us devotion to the created world; we behold creation in its eternal quickening, sprouting and ripening in veneration of the forces originating in the supersensible realm. In the second part, however, we look upwards in love towards the process of spiritualisation of the human soul, sensing with devotion the guiding powers of humanity. Spiritual science is then able to help us to grasp in thinking what devotion of will and love in feeling has guided us towards.

Rudolf Steiner however went still further. He asked what the outer expression of devotion is. 'We bend our knees, put our hands together and incline our head towards the object of our reverence.' This language of gesture is threefold: The bowed head, the folded hands and the bended knee. This threefoldness reappears in the table grace. We bend our knees towards the earth, for 'The plant-seeds are quickened in the night of the earth'. We fold our hands, for 'The green herbs are sprouting through the might of the air'. We bow our head in devotion, for 'The fruits are ripened by the power of the sun'.

And when human beings have learnt to perform these three gestures in devotion to the spiritual world, when they bend the knee in devotion to the divine-creative powers, when they have folded their hands and bowed their heads, they become bearers of light in the darkness of earth existence.

> By studying human nature, however, we learn that
> when our straight legs are stretched in strong, conscious
> action they do their best if they have first learnt to bend
> the knee where reverence is really due ... Hands which
> have learned to fold in reverence have received a force
> which can flow forth from the hand ... Bent in reverence
> ... a new force enters [the head] and the feeling this
> engenders is given back to the world.[7]

The soul – love and the good – will begin to quicken in the shrine of the heart of the human being standing upright upon the earth. The blessing of love for the other streams from the hands that have been folded in prayer. 'So ripens man's strength in the glory of God.' The human head, practising loving understanding, will bring to fulfilment the fruits of human potential ever ripening in the glory of God.

'Our' table grace is an everlasting practice of devotion, spoken in humility and love by the human being who strives to become a bearer of spirit. 'Love and humility are the appropriate guides to the realm of the unknown, and the educators of the soul from the intellectual soul to the consciousness soul.'

Publication details

The Prague lectures, *Cosmic and Earthly Nutrition,* were given in German in 1936.

A rough manuscript, slightly edited by Christoph Jensen, of *The Cultural Impulse in Agriculture,* the lectures given in English for farmers at Heathcot, Aberdeen in 1943, had been circulated among Camphill farmers, where they were known as the 'Milk Lectures.'

The Earthly and Cosmic Nutrition Streams, lectures given in English for doctors and farmers in Thornbury in 1953, and *The Meteorological Organs of the Earth and in the Human Being,* lectures given in English for farmers at Botton Village in 1958 were published in 1969 by the Biodynamic Farming and Gardening Association of North America as *Earth and Man,* edited by Carlo Pietzner, Alix Roth and Peter Roth.

'The Plant Seeds are Quickened' was first published in *Mitteilungen aus der anthroposophischen Arbeit in Deutschland,* Vol. 18, No. 1, Easter 1964.

Notes

A Note About this Volume

1   See Richard Steel, 'Motifs of the Social Mission in Karl König's Life'
     in König, *Becoming Human: A Social Task.*

Anthroposophic Nutritional Research

1   The results were published in the journal *Lebendige Erde,* 6/2007 and
     can also be found in the internet: *http://orgprints.org/3676/*

Cosmic and Earthly Nutrition: a Topical Question

1   Chyme is the semi-fluid mass into which food is converted by gastric
     secretion and which passes from the stomach into the small intestine.
2   Chyle is the milky fluid containing lymph and emulsified fat globules
     that forms from chyme in the small intestine, is absorbed by the
     lacteals, and reaches the bloodstream through the thoracic duct.
     Because of its emulsified fat content it is of milky consistency. The
     milky juice of plants is also known as chyle, as are high-fat lymph flu-
     ids that have a milky appearance.
3   Popp, *Biophotonen.* Popp proved that DNA is both receiver and trans-
     mitter of biophotonic rays. In a cell lacking DNA as a hereditary ves-
     sel, no biophotonic rays are measurable. Ensuing from this research
     various methods have been developed towards fields of practical
     application, for instance for quality control of foodstuffs, in diagnostic
     and therapeutic areas.
4   Steiner, *Agriculture,* pp. 260f.

Cosmic and Earthly Nutrition

1 Nutrition in General

1   König probably meant the observations that follow, also in the third
     lecture.

2   Since that time of course, travel, immigration and a global market have obscured this cultural differentiation.

3   Steiner mentioned such methods, for instance in *Illness and Therapy,* the lecture of April 18, 1921 about treatment for purulent ablation of the mucous membrane. Various contemporaries of König also wrote about milk injections; for instance, Odenthal and Kohl for the treatment of gonorrhoea by induced fever *(Dermatologische Zeitschrift,* No. 42, 1925).

4   The production of synthetic vitamin C was one of the first great technical breakthroughs in synthetic structuring with natural materials. In December 1933, two years after the discovery of vitamin C, Tadeus Reichenstein lodged a patent in Switzerland for the production of synthetic L-ascorbic acid. König certainly did not miss such developments.

5   There is no record of the conversations that took place before and after the lectures.

6   Apart from the many small glands in the oral mucosa there are three classifications of paired salivary glands: the parotid gland (near the ears) with starch-splitting enzymes; the glands inside the lower jaw (submandibular) and those underneath the tongue (sublingual), directly on the muscles of the mouth base, which produce mainly mucilage.

7   It seems that König has taken a radical stand here, possibly to make the importance of the process clear. In the other lectures this theme reappears in various ways. See also 'The breakdown of food and building up of individualised substance' in the introduction by Anita Pedersen.

8   Only in recent years has research (re)discovered the *abdominal brain,* which is the largest conflux of nerve cells outside the head; source of psychoactive substances that are to be seen in connection to our psychological constitution.

9   The neurologist Paul Julius Möbius (1853–1907) published an essay *(On the Physiological Idiocy of Women)* in 1900 that Rudolf Steiner obviously also quotes (without giving the name) in a lecture to workmen at the Goetheanum: 'The following happened with this professor: he measured brains and produced statistics showing his findings that women's brains are consistently smaller than men's. Because he was of the opinion that smaller brains have a smaller intelligence, he concluded that all women are less intelligent than men. ... But it was fashionable at that time to dissect the brains of famous men after they had died, and this was also done with the professor's brain. Lo and behold, this man's brain proved to be smaller than all the women's brains he had examined!' *(From Comets to Cocaine,* lecture of January 10, 1923).

10 Ilya Metchnikov (1845–1916), a Russian bacteriologist, received the Nobel Prize in 1908. Among other things he researched immunity and lactic acid bacteria.

11 Therese Neumann (1898–1962) was a German Catholic mystic and stigmatic, born in Konnersreuth, Bavaria. From 1923 until her death in 1962, she apparently consumed no food other than holy commun-

ion and claimed to have drunk no water from 1926 until her death. On this subject too, König was well ahead of his time. Recently 'light nourishment' has been researched in various places. One such person is the scientist Dr Michael Werner, who has lived since 2001 without solid and fluid nutrition (see Werner & Stöckli, *Life from Light*).

12 *Agriculture,* lecture of June 7, 1924.

13 *Agriculture,* lecture of June 16, 1924.

14 Angelus Silesius (1624–77), born Johannes Scheffler, German mystic poet and priest. The grace is from Silesius, *Der Cherubinische Wandersmann* (The Cherubinic Pilgrim).

2 Vegetarian Food or Meat?

1 *Physiology and Healing,* lecture of Dec 31, 1923, and *The Book of Revelation and the Work of the Priest,* lecture of Sep 13, 1924.

2 Chyle is the content of the lymphatic vessels that is transferred to the blood via the thoracic duct.

3 See also Steiner, *Introducing Anthroposophical Medicine,* lecture of March 29, 1920. This is further developed in Holtzapfel, *Human Organs.*

4 These statements refer back to Steiner's own qualitative method of observation for the effects of nutrition on the human being. Therefore the description of the potato being digested in the midbrain is not compatible to the usual scientific concepts of digestion but belongs to a more subtle view and is not provable by a materialistic approach.

5 In a lecture ('Ernährungsfragen im Lichte der Geisteswissenschaft') Steiner said the following and we quote it at length because this lecture has long been unavailable. 'The spiritual scientist's attitude must never agitate in favour of particular tendencies. He must be confident that when people have perceived the truth of what he says, they will then proceed to do the right thing. What I have to say therefore does not recommend one course as opposed to another, and anyone who assumes that it does, will misunderstand it completely. Merely the facts will be stated. ... Even though a vegetarian diet might indeed be the correct one for some people purely for reasons of health, the health of others might be ruined by it. I am speaking here of human nature in general, of course, but it must of course be considered individually. ... Today, an excess of meat in the diet naturally brings its corresponding results. ... The soul will become more externally oriented, more susceptible to and bound up with the external world. If people take their nourishment from the realm of plants, however, they become more independent and more inclined to develop inwardly. They become master over their whole being.

6 Steiner, *Original Impulses for the Science of the Spirit,* lecture of Oct 22, 1906.

7 Neurologists have recently discovered that the brain can indeed be developed and formed by the way one thinks.

8 Steiner gave clear indications as to the effects of meat or vegetarian diet on the soul life of the human being, widening this out to take in the methods of feeding animals and in a certain sense foreseeing the BSE (mad cow disease) catastrophe of the 1980s (*From Comets to Cocaine,* lecture of Jan 13, 1923).

9 Steiner describes this process a number of times, for instance in *From Crystals to Crocodiles* (lecture of Aug 9, 1922), and in *Harmony of the Creative Word* (lecture of Oct 28, 1923). König worked intensely on the questions of the glands, writing 'Das Problem der inneren Sekretion' for the journal of the Medical Section *Natura* in 1928 (Vol.2/7), and 'Meditations on the Endocrine Glands' for the *Golden Blade* (1952/3).

3 Childhood and Infant Nutrition

1 At that time it was not yet generally so well known how harmful alcohol is for children and youngsters.

2 Today it is more usual to recommend supplementary substances from the fifth month as prevention of allergies.

3 Now lactose and yoghurt are recommended that were not as easily available then, whereas malt is no longer so well known today. Again, due to the increase in allergies one needs to be careful with citrus juices as a child can react with sores.

4 This reference could not be found. However, in *Foundations of Esotericism,* Steiner stated the following: 'A condition arose when milk became the general nourishment for mankind, and then the condition when nourishment was provided by the mother's milk. Before the time when milk was imbibed from Nature, there was an age in which the earth was still united with the sun. There then existed a sun nourishment. Just as milk has remained from the moon, products have also remained which gained their maturity from the sun. Everything irradiated with sunlight, blossoms and fruits of the plants, belongs to the sun. Formerly their growth inclined towards the centre of the earth when it was united with the sun. They planted themselves into the sun with their blossoms. When the earth separated from the sun they retained their old character: they again turned their blossoms towards the sun. Man is the plant in reverse. That part of the plant which grows above the earth has the same relationship to the sun as milk has to the moon; is therefore sun-food. Side by side with milk nourishment there arose a kind of plant nourishment, namely from the upper parts of the plant. This was the second form of human food.' (lecture of Nov 4, 1905).

5 König evidently saw this as a general principle, but as he again and again warns, nothing should be taken dogmatically and implemented

in that way, but rather an individual decision should be made according to the constitution of the particular child. At present in anthroposophical nutritional research carrots are often recommended as first supplementary food, but also here an understanding of the individual constitution is basis for the decision. The question remains open whether today's situation calls for a different step, or whether König's observations perhaps offer a new approach to general aspects in respect to modern developments.

An indication Steiner made may help: 'The part of the human being that is related to the whole earth is the head. Not the feet, but actually the head. When the human being starts to be an earthly being in the womb, he has at first almost nothing but a head. He begins with his head. His head takes the shape of the whole cosmos and the shape of the earth. And the head particularly needs minerals. For it is from the head that the forces go out that fill the human body with bones, for instance. Everything that makes a human being solid is the result of the way the head has been formed. While the head itself is still soft, as in the womb, it cannot form bones properly. But as it becomes harder and harder itself, it passes to the body the forces by which both man and animal are able to form their solid parts, particularly their bones. You can see from this that we need roots. They are related to the earth and contain minerals. We need the minerals for bone-building. Bones consist of calcium carbonate, calcium phosphate; those are minerals. So you can see that the human being needs roots in order to strengthen his head. (*From Sunspots to Strawberries*, lecture of July 31, 1924, p. 84).

6   Sago is a starch product of the sago palm or of manioc. Today it is more usual to use wholemeal flour.

7   König's deliberations about the different constitutional types of children follow the descriptions Rudolf Steiner made during the Curative Education course (*Education for Special Needs,* lecture of June 30) and in the *Faculty Meetings* with teachers on Feb 6, 1923. In all these descriptions there is a common theme of the connection between the constitution and nutrition. This is certainly why König uses these examples here. In the context of the lecture it was not possible for him to go into more detail, therefore he has attempted to deal with the rather complex matter in a short and lively, imaginative way. It is helpful to expand this simplified and generalised passage by referring back to the original lectures by Rudolf Steiner.

8   For instance in *The Education of the Child* and particularly in *Foundations of Human Experience,* the lectures given at the founding of the first Waldorf School.

9   A Mrs Mittak had composed several temperament-specific menus. There seems to have been practical examples of dietary possibilities.

4 Special Diets

1 During his time in Silesia König gave regular talks in Prague and visited patients there. On April 22, 1933 he had spoken about nutrition and healing; only his short notes remain (Karl König Archive, Aberdeen).

2 Ragnar Berg (1873–1956), a Swedish biochemist and nutritionist, was the founder of the theory of acid-base balance and set up the postulation in 1912 that illness often occurs through hyperacidity.

3 *Harmony of the Creative Word,* lecture of Nov 10, 1923.

4 Johann Schroth (1798–1856) devised natural cures for purification and detoxification of the body, and to reduce weight.

5 Max Gerson (1881–1959) became famous in the 1920s for his saltless, fresh food based diet that was supposedly good against tuberculosis and cancer. At the time and also today it is controversial because of its high dosages of codliver oil with phosphorus, which led to a positive weight gain for TB-patients but also carried a number of side effects. Prince Charles once received negative publicity for recommending Gerson's treatment for cancer patients (*The Guardian,* 26th June 2004), whereas Albert Schweizer, whose wife was supposedly cured of TB by Gerson, called him 'one of the greatest geniuses in the history of medicine.' (Straus, *Dr Max Gerson)*

The Cultural Impulse of Agriculture

1 Milk and Blood

1 We have left this quote in although we have until now not been able to identify the source. König usually only had the German lecture cycles and took them to a lecture, translating freely.

2 The source of this quote could not be found. A 1984 study showed that 540 litres of blood needs to flow through the milk glands of a cow for it to produce one litre of milk (Kielwein, *Leitfaden der Milchkunde)*

3 Ernst Lehrs had given 2 lectures, 'Natural Science and Spiritual Science' at this conference. Luke Howard (1772–1864), English pharmacist and hobby meteorologist, in 1882 developed the method of cloud classification still used today.

4 *From Sunspots to Strawberries,* lecture of June 30 1924.

5 *Mystery Knowledge and Mystery Centres,* lecture of Dec 1, 1923.

6 Carl Gustav Carus (1789–1869) German physiologist and painter. His book, *Grundzüge der vergleichenden Anatomie und Physiologie,* was first printed in 1828.

7 Ernest Henry Starling (1866–1927) English physiologist. *Principles of Human Physiology,* p. 1196.

2 Faeces and the Brain

1 *Introducing Anthroposophical Medicine,* March 24, 1920, p. 64.
2 The source of this quote as not been found. The studies about this marsupial were by the American surgeon, biologist and theosophist Samuel Elliot Cues, *On the Osteology and Mythology of* Didelphys virginiana.
3 It represents about 50% of the solids in the faeces but only about 10% of the faeces altogether.
4 Apart from the intestinal juices there are also enzymes, bacteria of the enteric flora and intestinal cells, meaning that the largest part of the faeces consists indeed of intestinal juices – otherwise there are only left-overs of dietary fibres.
5 Steiner, *Agricultural,* lecture of June 16, 1924.
6 Today one is able to trace small amounts of albumin particles and sugar.

3 The Rain of Cosmic Nutrition

1 Therese Neumann (1898–1962) was a Catholic mystic and stigmatic. From 1923 until her death in 1962, she apparently consumed no food other than holy communion and claimed to have drunk no water from 1926 until her death.
2 Recently 'light nourishment' has been researched in various places. One such person is the scientist Dr Michael Werner, who has lived since 2001 without solid and fluid nutrition (see Werner & Stöckli, *Life from Light*).
3 *Agriculture,* lecture of June 12, 1924.
4 There are various descriptions of horns and antlers in König's *Social Farming.*
5 To make biodynamic yarrow and horn silica preparations a stag's bladder and a cow's horn are used, as described thoroughly in König's *Social Farming.*
6 In this case drinkable alcohol is not meant but the ethyl traces found during the metabolic processes; for instance acetyl coenzyme A being produced during the breakdown of carbohydrates and in the fatty acid oxidation.

Earthly and Cosmic Nutritional Streams in Human Beings and Plants

1 The Contrast Between the Senses and Digestion

1 Steiner said: 'What is the brain mass, actually? The substance of the brain is simply intestinal content taken as far as possible, whereas premature brain deposits pass out through the intestines. The contents of the intestine, as regards their processes, are very much related to the contents

of the brain. It would be crass to say that what is present in the brain is simply a more highly developed manure pile, but objectively this is quite correct. The manure is transformed by means of the organic process into the noble substance of the brain, where it becomes the basis for development of the ego.' Steiner, *Agriculture,* lecture of June 16, 1924, p. 157.

2 *Broken Vessels,* lecture of Sep 14, 1924.

3 Steiner, *Mensch und Welt,* lecture of Oct 31, 1923.

4 The 'three semi-circular canals' are the horizontal semicircular canal (also known as the lateral semicircular canal), the superior semicircular canal (also known as the anterior semicircular canal), and the posterior semicircular canal of the inner ear. See also the lectures 'Meteorological Organs,' later in this volume.

5 For instance, in *The Foundations of Human Experience,* lecture of Aug 21, 1919.

6 Both series of lectures are in Steiner, *A Psychology of Body, Soul and Spirit.*

7 The idea of the threefold human being was first developed in 1917 in *The Riddles of the Soul.*

8 Today this condition is more acute with the virtual reality of computer games and the internet.

9 Johannes Peter Müller (1801–54), physiologist and anatomist. He placed physiology next to philosophy because he believed that empirically gained facts need to be understood and synthesised through philosophical thought. In 1826 his voluminous study about comparative physiology of the sense of sight *(Zur vergleichenden Physiologie des Gesichtssinnes)* containing much material about the sight of animals and humans which was new for his times. There were, for instance, observations of the composite eyes of insects and crabs, and analytic descriptions of the human gaze and its forms of expression. It was considered to be a historic achievement that he recognised each individual sensory system to react to its own type of stimulus in its own fashion – or as Müller put it: answering with its own specific energy. Also in 1826 he published a book about 'fantastic phenomena of sight' *(Über die phantastischen Gesichtserscheinungen),* in which he showed how the sensory system of sight reacts towards internal as well as external stimuli; for instance through mental pictures and imagination. This theory of internal sense stimuli is still valid in science today and Müller is considered to be one of those who changed the world during the nineteenth century, moving medicine on from the romantic natural philosophical mode to being based on modern natural science. He influenced particularly Jakob Henle, Theodor Schwann, Rudolf Virchow, Hermann von Helmholtz and Emil du Bois-Reymond.

10 Immoral forces have not gone through the process of digestion. This theme comes up again in the discussion following the fourth lecture (p. 231).

2 Nutrition in Digestion and the Senses

1 *Introducing Anthroposophical Medicine,* lecture of April 3, 1920.
2 *From Elephants to Einstein* (Jan 23, 1924) and *Mensch und Welt* (Oct 20, 1923).
3 *Human Evolution,* lecture of Aug 25, 1918.
4 The German physician Wilhelm Heinrich Schüssler (1821–98) was originally a supporter of homeopathy, but then developed his own theory of 12 biochemic cell salts designed to help retain different minerals from nutrition and to stimulate various bodily functions. Samuel Hahnemann (1755–1843) was the founder of homoeopathy; see also König, *At the Threshold of the Modern Age.*
5 Probably the connection between anaemia and iron metabolism is meant. Around this time (1953) König began to study this theme extensively, discovering a thesis in 1955 describing four main 'tongue types', and took the opportunity to write about the four blood-types in this context for the journal *Beiträge zur Erweiterung der Heilkunst,* (Nov/Dec 1956).
6 Steiner, *The Universe, Earth and Man,* lecture of Aug 6, 1908.
7 At that time one spoke of the 'combustion' of carbohydrates and fats within the cell. The products of this process are mineral substances (ash) and light.
8 König often studied the endocrine glands. In this context his essay 'Meditations on the Endocrine Glands' *(The Golden Blade,* 1952) is particularly pertinent.

3 Silica and Calcium

1 *Foundations of Human Experience,* lecture of Aug 22, 1919.
2 These substances (nitrogen, hydrogen, carbon, sulphur, phosphorus) in contrast to the others, build the nutrients albumin, fat and carbohydrates.
3 Preparation 505 in Steiner, *Agriculture Course.* See also 'The Sheaths of the Preparations' in König, *Social Farming.*
4 *Das Miterleben des Jahreslaufes,* lecture of Oct 7, 1923.
5 *Agriculture,* lecture of June 13, 1924. Steiner indicates that this begins to happen through applying the biodynamic preparations. Also see the discussion with König following his lecture.
6 The calcium within the blood is important for the process of coagulation.
7 *Das Miterleben des Jahreslaufes,* lecture of Oct 13, 1923.
8 'The Michael Imagination' in *The Archangel Michael,* lecture of Oct 5, 1923.
9 *Agriculture,* lecture of June 11, 1924.
10 Steiner, *From Crystals to Crocodiles,* lecture of Sep 23, 1922.
11 Vermeulen describes the role of silica in the plant and in the human

body in a similar way, and also remarks on the relatively high concentration in the lens of the eye. For concentration in the umbilical cord, see also Hecht, 'Das essenzielle Spurenelement Silizium' in *Naturmineralien.*

12 König was referring to a statement he made in earlier lectures in 1947. See 'The sheaths of the Preparations' in *Social Farming.*

13 It has since been proved that the use of Preparation 500 on grazing pastures significantly reduces bloating. See Don Rathbone, 'Biodynamic Farming,' in *Biodynamic Growing* Victoria, Australia 1992.

4 The Endocrine Glands

1 Steiner, *Becoming the Archangel Michael's Companions,* lecture of Oct, 3, 1922.

2 The connection of hormones to these organs appears to be the result of Karl König's own research.

3 At that time the term was still used, also officially in diagnostics, for persons with an IQ of less than 20–30%.

4 This was certainly more the case at that time. Today there is generally a greater degree of differentiation and individualisation, although König's observation is still principally valid. He studied these phenomena widely at the time, and wrote some essays, particularly *Der Mongolismus.*

5 This refers to myasthenia gravis, an auto-immune condition of the Thymus gland.

6 Cortisone was discovered in 1935, and produced from 1949.

7 'Meditations on the Endocrine Glands' in *The Golden Blade,* 1952.

8 Rainer Maria Rilke (1875–1926), German poet, died of leukemia. This disease, first described by Rudolf Virchow in 1845, entails a strong overproduction of white blood-corpuscles (leucocytes; König calls them 'white lymph').

9 Gladstone & Wakely, *The Pineal Organ.*

The Meteorological Organs

1 Introduction

1 Maurice Wood (1884–1960) started the first bio-dynamic farm in Britain, in Huby near Leeds in 1929. He helped George Adams to translate Rudolf Steiner's Agriculture Course in 1930. His mill (Huby Mill) was the first meeting place of the British biodynamic movement.

2 *Therapeutic Insights,* lecture of July 1, 1921.

3 Adolf Portmann (1897–1982), Swiss zoologist. His work was often interdisciplinary compromising sociological and philosophical aspects

of life of animals and humans. He was influenced particularly by Jakob von Uexküll, whose lectures also König had visited in Vienna. Portmann wrote *Animals as Social Beings* in 1953 (English 1961) and *Zoologie und das neue Bild des Menschen,* 1956.

4 *Introducing Anthroposophical Medicine,* lecture of March 29, 1920.

5 Persorption is the non re-absorbing ingestion of microparticles in the intestinal wall.

6 In the previous lectures in this volume König spoke more about this theme, particularly in the first Prague lecture. A certain amount of permeation can be found, especially through more exact measurements that are possible today. For König, however, it is more important to understand the process of breaking down substance and 'rebuilding' on the other side of the intestinal wall.

7 In *Mystery Knowledge and Mystery Centres.*

2 The Lung

1 *Introducing Anthroposophical Medicine,* lecture of March 29, 1920.

2 *Harmony of the Creative Word;* also in *A Modern Art of Education,* lecture of Aug 13, 1923.

3 Eugen Kolisko (1893–1939), physician and teacher at the first Waldorf School in Stuttgart; he was from Vienna, where he knew König during his youth and introduced him to anthroposophy. He wrote *The Twelve Groups of Animals.*

4 Inhaling on average 18 times per minute is 1080 in the hour, or 25920 per day. The Platonic Year is the time taken for the vernal equinox to move round the zodiac. See also Steiner, *Cosmic and Human Metamorphosis,* lecture of Feb 13, 1917.

5 Steiner spoke in more detail of this in *Supersensible Knowledge,* lecture of Oct 25, 1906.

6 Steiner, *Therapeutic Insights,* lecture of July 3, 1921.

3 The Spheres Surrounding the Earth

1 Today it is known that the temperature in the ozone layers rises from below $-50°$ to $0°C$ ($-60°$ to $32°F$). Not until the mesosphere does the temperature rise above $0°C$. The actual warmth layer is the thermosphere (or ionosphere) at a height of 85 km (55 mi). There the temperatures can reach $2500°C$ ($4500°F$), higher than König had thought.

2 Wachsmuth, *The Etheric Formative Forces in Cosmos, Earth and Man,* New York 1932 (original German 1924).

3 Currently the ionosphere is described in various layers. D layer: 60–90 km (40–55 mi); E-layer: 90–120 km (55–75 mi); F1 and F2 layers: 200–500 km (125–300 miles). In the F-layers the gaseous particles are ionised by the sunrays, facilitating high frequency radio communications over long distances.

4   *Introducing Anthroposophical Medicine,* lecture of March 29, 1920.
5   *Spirit as Sculptor of the Human Organism,* lectures of Oct 20, 22 and 23,
    1922; and *Physiology and Healing,* lectures of Oct 26, 27 and 28, 1922.
6   *Education for Special Needs,* lecture of July 1, 1924.
7   Current theory is that the fats pass into the lymph, other substances
    into the blood.
8   There were two studies that went in this direction. Linus Pauling
    received the Nobel Prize for Chemistry in 1954 for his work on the
    structure of proteins. Arne Tiselius received the Nobel Prize for
    Chemistry in 1948 for research in electrophoresis and adsorption
    analysis, especially for his discoveries concerning the complex nature
    of the serum proteins.

4 The Liver

1   Steiner, *Four Mystery Dramas: The Portal of Initiation,* Scene 5, pp. 99f.
2   Steiner, *Colour.*
3   At this point the transcribed text becomes very scanty and inadequate,
    obscuring its meaning. In the rest of the paragraph James Dyson has
    attempted to reconstruct what Dr König was trying to convey.
4   Medical physiology distinguishes between the absorption of lipids
    (fats), which appear to be selectively absorbed into the lacteals (lym-
    phatic capillaries), as micelles, and the absorption of simple carbo-
    hydrates and amino acids into the intestinal blood capillaries of the
    portal venous system. (I am not aware that Rudolf Steiner made this
    particular distinction, nor that it was known during his lifetime. This
    makes the matter under consideration somewhat more complex, but
    does not necessarily alter Steiner's fundamental hypothesis. James
    Dyson.)
5   Recent estimates of the liver's blood flow suggest 1.2 litres/minute
    (1.25 quarts/minute).
6   See 'The Sheaths of the Preparations' in König, *Social Farming.*
7   This is known as the liver and gall bladder rhythm.
8   This probably refers to hepatitis B which can be contracted epidemi-
    cally by means of bodily fluids, especially blood.
9   The viruses responsible for jaundice and polio are similar although
    the diseases they cause are completely different.
10 At that time one was not yet able to distinguish between viral hepati-
    tis B and the bacterial form hepatitis A. Bacterial hepatitis A can even
    be contracted through contaminated foodstuffs.
11 *Spirit as Sculptor of the Human Organism,* particularly the lecture of Oct
    22, 1922.
12 *Therapeutic Insights,* lecture of July 2, 1921.
13 *Mensch und Welt,* lecture of Oct 13, 1923.
14 *Secret Brotherhoods,* lecture of Nov 16, 1917.

15 Today ATP (adenosine triphosphate) is reckoned as a source of energy. It is derived from carbohydrates and fats with the help of oxygen.

16 *The Presence of the Dead,* lecture of May 12, 1914, and *Education for Adolescence,* lecture of June 12, 1921.

17 Steiner, *Agriculture,* lecture of June 11, 1924, pp. 58f.

5 The Kidney

1 *Agriculture,* lecture of June 11, 1924.

2 Probably *Spirit as Sculptor of the Human Organism*, lecture of Oct 20, 1922.

3 Bowman's capsule is a cup-shaped sac forming the beginning of the tubular component of a nephron, the functional unit of a kidney. It performs the first step in the filtration of blood, eventually leading to the formation of the urine. A system of arteriolar capillaries forming a single structural component and called a glomerulus is enclosed by Bowman's capsule through a process of invagination. Fluids from blood capillaries within each glomerulus pass over into the inner sac or lumen of Bowman's capsule – a process driven by pressurised filtration, which forms the primary urine or glomerular filtrate at the rate of 170 litres per 24 hours. This is then processed further by active metabolic processes within the subsequent course of each nephron, eventually forming urine. This processing involves fluid re-absorption of approximately 168 litres per 24 hours as well as complex, highly selective reabsorption of minerals and organic compounds, generally against a concentration gradient, involving a great deal of metabolic energy and oxygen.

4 Renin and its effect on blood pressure were first identified at the end of the nineteenth century. It is an enzyme secreted by specialised kidney cells in the juxtaglomerular apparatus. A year before this lecture was given, its action in the conversion of angiotensinogen into angiotensin was established after decades of intensive research, mainly in South America and the USA. Subsequently this knowledge provided the basis for the development of several generations of drugs for the treatment of hypertension (initially the ACE inhibitors). These have now been in routine use in general medicine for several decades. Renin is secreted directly into the bloodstream like a hormone when either blood pressure, blood volume or the sodium content of the blood is low. The liver, the lung as well as the adrenal cortex are now known to be involved in the cascade of metabolic processes for which it is the main catalyst. The fact that the mode of action of renin was only beginning to be unravelled when König originally gave this lecture suggests his keen awareness of the latest scientific developments.

5 *Physiology and Healing,* lecture of Oct 27, 1922, p. 81.

6 *Spirit as Sculptor of the Human Organism*, lecture of Oct 23, 1922.

7 Gisbert Husemann (1907–97) was a physician and friend of Karl König. He was co-founder of the Association of Anthroposophical Physicians in Germany and editor of the journal *Beiträge zu einer Erweiterung der Heilkunst* for which König wrote many articles. Husemann's speciality was the connection between medicine and geology.

8 *Introducing Anthroposophical Medicine,* lecture of March 31, 1920, and *Physiology and Healing,* lecture of April 7, 1920.

9 König develops this theme in his *The Calendar of the Soul: A Commentary.* There he shows the sequence of verses can be seen in the form of a lemniscate, as is the structure of the year itself. Summer and winter are at opposite poles, while the spring and autumn stand at the crossing point, like a central heart.

10 Steiner, *Introducing Anthroposophical Medicine,* lecture of March 31, 1920.

11 *Introducing Anthroposophical Medicine,* lecture of March 31, 1920.

12 *From Beetroot to Buddhism,* lecture of June 4, 1924.

13 Steiner described this in *Man in the Light of Occultism, Philosophy and Theosophy.*

6 The Heart

1 Steiner spoke of the spleen in *An Occult Physiology.* Lili Kolisko (1889–1976) worked with Rudolf Steiner doing scientific research following his indications. In 1922 she published a study about the spleen, *Milzfunktion und Plättchenfrage.* She was the wife of Eugen Kolisko, a close friend of König's. The Koliskos emigrated to England in 1934. In old age she said of herself, 'Take the work on the spleen (1922) and follow through to the lead (1952) then you have my biography.'

2 *The Cycle of the Year,* lecture of Sep 30, 1923.

3 Steiner described this: 'Regarding the other organs, I have told you that the out-flowing of organic forces can become hallucinatory life, especially what is pressed out of the liver system. If the heart presses out its contents, however, this is really a system of forces, pushed out and brought into consciousness, that call forth in the next incarnation that strange inclination to live out one's karma. If one observes how karma works itself out, it may be said from the human side that this living out of karma can only be described as a kind of hunger and its satisfaction.' *(Therapeutic Insights,* lecture of July 2, 1921).

4 *Vergangenheits- und Zukunftsimpulse,* lecture of April 5, 1919.

5 Pietism was a movement within Lutheranism that began in the late seventeenth century and reached its zenith in the mid-eighteenth century. John (1703–91) and Charles (1709–88) Wesley founded the Methodist Church after affiliating themselves to the Herrnhut (Moravian) Brotherhood.

6 *The Human Soul in Relation to World Evolution,* lecture of May 26, 1922 (that lecture also published as 'The Human Heart' in *The Golden Blade* 1976).

7 Friedrich Rittelmeyer (1872–1938) one of the founders of the Christian Community.

8 Emanuel Swedenborg (1688–1772). See Steiner, *Karmic Relationships,* Vol. 8, lecture of August 24, 1924.

9 *The Kingdom of Childhood,* lecture series in August 1924.

10 *Mensch und Welt,* lecture of Oct 20, 1923.

11 *First Scientific Lecture-Course,* lecture of Jan 2, 1920.

12 The World Conference for Spiritual Science and its Practical Applications, London, July 23 and 24, 1928. This was König's first connection to the English-speaking world. He travelled there with Ita Wegman, gave a talk about the origin of man and embryology.

13 In fact Daniel Dunlop was very deeply and directly involved in the initiative behind this conference, and particularly in its practical preparation.

Two Essays

The Relation of Intestine and Brain

1 *Introducing Anthroposophical Medicine,* lecture of March 24, 1920, p. 64.

2 *Agriculture,* lecture of June 16, 1924, pp. 155, 157.

The Plant-Seeds Are Quickened

1 The verses of the *Soul Calendar* in this essay are from A.C. Harwood's translation *(The Meditative Year).*

2 These examples are from Heiler, *Das Gebet.*

3 From Silesius, *Der Cherubinische Wandersmann* (The Cherubinic Pilgrim).

4 There is no version of this in Steiner's handwriting, so it is not certain that he is the author.

5 *Transforming the Soul,* lecture of Oct 28, 1909, p. 94.

6 *Transforming the Soul,* lecture of Oct 28, 1909, p. 85.

7 *Transforming the Soul,* lecture of Oct 28, 1909, pp. 91f.

Bibliography

Carus, Carl Gustav, *Grundzüge der vergleichenden Anatomie und Physiologie*, first printed in 1828.

Cues, Samuel Elliot, *On the Osteology and Mythology of* Didelphys virginiana, Boston 1872.

Gladstone, R.I., and Wakely, C.P.G. *The Pineal Organ*, London 1940.

Hauschka, Rudolf, *The Nature of Substance: Spirit and Matter*, Rudolf Steiner Press, UK 2008.

—, *Nutrition: A Holistic Approach*, Rudolf Steiner Press, UK 2008.

Hecht, Karl & Hecht-Savoley, Elena, *Naturmineralien, Regulation, Gesundheit*, Schribi, Berlin 2005.

Heiler, Friedrich, *Das Gebet*, Munich 1921.

Holtzapfel, Walter, *Human Organs – Their Functional and Psychological Significance: Liver, Lung, Kidney, Heart*, Floris Books, 2013.

Howard, Luke, *The Modification of Clouds*, London 1803.

Kielwein, Gerhard, *Leitfaden der Milchkunde*, Berlin 1984.

Kolisko, Eugen, *The Twelve Groups of Animals*, Kolisko Archive 1977.

Kolisko, Lili, *Milzfunktion und Plättchenfrage*, Stuttgart 1922.

König, Karl, *At the Threshold of the Modern Age*, Floris Books, 2011.

—, *Becoming Human: A Social Task*, Floris Books, 2011.

—, *The Calendar of the Soul: A Commentary*, Floris Books, 2010.

—, *Der Mongolismus*, Hippokrates, Stuttgart 1959.

—, *Social Farming*, Floris Books 2014.

Mann, Thomas, *The Magic Mountain*, Knopf, New York 1927.

Müller, Johannes Peter, *Über die phantastischen Gesichtserscheinungen*, 1826.

—, *Zur vergleichenden Physiologie des Gesichtssinnes*, 1826.

Popp, F.A., *Biophotonen. Neue Horizonte in der Medizin: Von den Grundlagen zur Biophotonik*, Karl Haug 2006.

Portmann, Adolf, *Animals as Social Beings*, 1961

—, *Zoologie und das neue Bild des Menschen*, 1956.

Schmidt, Gerhard, *The Dynamics of Nutrition*, Biodynamic Association, USA 1980.

—, *The Essentials of Nutrition*, Biodynamic Association, USA 1987.

Selg, Peter, *Ita Wegman and Karl König*, Floris Books 2009.

Simonis, Werner Christian, *Die Ernährung des Menschen*, Freies Geistesleben, Stuttgart 1960.

—, *Milch und Honig,* Freies Geistesleben, Stuttgart 1965.

Starling, Ernest Henry, *Principles of Human Physiology,* 1912.

Steiner, Rudolf. Volume Nos refer to the Collected Works (CW), or to the German Gesamtausgabe (GA).

—, *Agriculture Course: The Birth of the Biodynamic Method* (CW 327) Rudolf Steiner Press, UK 2004 (also published as *Agriculture).*

—, *Agriculture: Spiritual Foundations for the Renewal of Agriculture* (CW 327) Biodynamic Association of North America 1993. (also published as *Agriculture Course).*

—, *The Archangel Michael: His Mission and Ours,* Anthroposophic Press, USA 1994.

—, *Becoming the Archangel Michael's Companions* (CW 217) SteinerBooks, USA 2007.

—, *The Book of Revelation and the Work of the Priest* (CW 346) Rudolf Steiner Press, UK 1999.

—, *Broken Vessels: the Spiritual Structure of Human Frailty* (CW 318) SteinerBooks, USA 2002.

—, *The Christ Impulse and the Development of Ego-Consciousness* (CW 116) Rudolf Steiner Press, UK 2014.

—, *Colour,* Rudolf Steiner Press, UK 1997.

—, *Cosmic and Human Metamorphosis* (CW 175) SteinerBooks, USA 2012.

—, *The Cycle of the Year* (CW 223) Anthroposophic Press, USA 1984.

—, *Education for Adolescents* (CW 302) Anthroposophic Press, USA 1996.

—, *Education for Special Needs: The Curative Education Course* (CW 317) Rudolf Steiner Press, UK 2014.

—, *The Education of the Child,* Anthroposophic Press, USA 1996.

—, 'Ernährungsfragen im Lichte der Geisteswissenschaft' (Jan 8, 1909) in *Das Goetheanum,* No. 47 & 48, Vol 14, 1935.

— with Ita Wegman, *Extending Practical Medicine* (CW 27) Rudolf Steiner Press, UK 1997.

—, *Faculty Meetings with Rudolf Steiner* (CW 300) 2 vols. Anthroposophic Press, USA 1998.

—, *The Festivals and Their Meaning,* Rudolf Steiner Press, UK 1996.

—, *First Scientific Lecture-Course: Light Course* (CW 320) Goethean Science Foundation, UK 1977.

—, *Foundations of Esotericism* (CW 93a) Rudolf Steiner Press, UK 1983.

—, *The Foundations of Human Experience* (CW 293) Anthroposophic Press, USA 1996.

—, *Four Mystery Dramas* (CW 14) SteinerBooks, USA 2014.

—, *From Beetroot to Buddhism* (CW 354) Rudolf Steiner Press, UK 1999.

—, *From Comets to Cocaine* (CW 348) Rudolf Steiner Press, UK 2002.

—, *From Crystals to Crocodiles ... Answers to Questions* (CW 347) Rudolf Steiner Press, UK 2002.

—, *From Limestone to Lucifer* (CW 349) Rudolf Steiner Press, UK 2000.

—, *From Sunspots to Strawberries* (CW 354) Rudolf Steiner Press, UK 2002.

—, *Harmony of the Creative Word: the Human Being and the Elemental, Animal, Plant and Mineral Kingdoms* (CW 230) Rudolf Steiner Press, UK 2002.

—, *Human Evolution: A Spiritual-Scientific Quest* (CW 183) Rudolf Steiner Press, UK 2014.

—, *The Human Soul in Relation to World Evolution* (CW 212) Anthroposophic Press, USA 1970.

—, *Illness and Therapy: Spiritual-Scientific Aspects of Healing* (CW 313) Rudolf Steiner Press, UK 2013.

—, *Introducing Anthroposophical Medicine* (CW 312) SteinerBooks, USA 2010.

—, *Karmic Relationships: Esoteric Studies,* Volume 8 (CW 240) Rudolf Steiner Press, UK 1995.

—, *The Kingdom of Childhood* (CW 311) Anthroposophic Press, USA 1995.

—, *Man in the Light of Occultism, Philosophy and Theosophy* (CW 137) Rudolf Steiner Press, UK 1964.

—, *The Meditative Year,* Tr. A.C. Harwood, Rudolf Steiner Press, UK 1970.

—, *Mensch und Welt: das Wirken des Geistes in der Natur* (GA 351) Dornach 1999.

—, *Das Miterleben des Jahreslaufes in vier kosmischen Imaginationen* (GA 229) Dornach 1999.

—, *A Modern Art of Education* (CW 307) SteinerBooks, USA 2000.

—, *Mystery Knowledge and Mystery Centres* (CW 232) Rudolf Steiner Press, UK 2013.

—, *An Occult Physiology* (CW 128) Rudolf Steiner Press, UK 2005.

—, *Original Impulses for the Science of the Spirit* (CW 96) Completion Press, Australia 2001.

—, *Physiology and Healing: Treatment, Therapy and Hygiene* (CW 314) Rudolf Steiner Press, UK 2013.

—, *The Presence of the Dead on the Spiritual Path* (CW 154) Anthroposophic Press, USA 1990.

—, *A Psychology of Body, Soul and Spirit: Anthroposophy, Psychosophy, Pneumatosophy* (CW 115) Anthroposophic Press, USA 1999.

—, *The Riddles of the Soul* (CW 21) Mercury Press, USA 1996.

—, *Secret Brotherhoods and the Mystery of the Human Double* (CW 178) Rudolf Steiner Press, UK 2004.

—, *Spirit as Sculptor of the Human Organism* (CW 218) Rudolf Steiner Press, UK 2014.

—, *Supersensible Knowledge* (CW 55) Anthroposophic Press, USA 1988.

—, *Therapeutic Insights: Earthly and Cosmic Laws* (CW 205) Mercury Press, USA 1984.

—, *Transforming the Soul,* Vol. 1 (CW 58) Rudolf Steiner Press, UK 2005.

—, *The Universe, Earth and Man* (CW 105) Rudolf Steiner Press, UK 1987.

—, *Vergangenheits- und Zukunftsimpulse im Sozialen Geschehen: die geistigen Hintergründe der sozialen Frage* (GA 190) Dornach 1980.

Straus, Howard, *Dr Max Gerson: Healing the Hopeless,* Kingston, Ontario, Canada: Quarry Books, 2001

Strindberg, August, *En blå bok,* 1913. Translated into English by Claud Field as *Zones of the Spirit.*

Vermeulen, Frans, *Homöopathische Substanzen,* Sonntag, Stuttgart 2004.

Wachsmuth, Guenther, *The Etheric Formative Forces in Cosmos, Earth and Man,* New York 1932.

Werner, Michael and Stöckli, Thomas, *Life from Light,* Clairview, 2007.

Wolf, E. *Aschen-Analysen von land- und forstwirtschaftilichen Produkten,* Berlin, 1871, 1880.

Index

Karl König's collected works are being published in English by Floris Books, Edinburgh and in German by Verlag Freies Geistesleben, Stuttgart. They are issued by the Karl König Archive, Aberdeen in co-operation with the Ita Wegman Institute for Basic Research into Anthroposophy, Arlesheim. They seek to encompass the entire, wide-ranging literary estate of Karl König, including his books, essays, manuscripts, lectures, diaries, notebooks, his extensive correspondence and his artistic works. The publications will fall into twelve subjects.

The aim is to open up König's work in a systematic way and make it accessible. This work is supported by many people in different countries.

Overview of Karl König Archive subjects

Medicine and study of the human being
Curative education and social therapy
Psychology and education
Agriculture and science
Social questions
The Camphill movement
Christianity and the festivals
Anthroposophy
Spiritual development
History and biographies
Artistic and literary works
Karl König's biography

Karl König Archive
Camphill House
Milltimber
Aberdeen AB13 0AN
United Kingdom
www.karl-koenig-archive.net
aberdeen@karl-koenig-archive.net

Ita Wegman Institute for Basic
    Research into Anthroposophy
Pfeffingerweg 1a
4144 Arlesheim
Switzerland
www.wegmaninstitut.ch
koenigarchiv@wegmaninstitut.ch

The Karl König Archive